Home life:

a code of practice for residential care

Dixon-Carter
Easter Balnabaan
Drumnadrochit
Inverness-shire IV3 6UK
Tel: Drumnadrochit (04562) 310

D0277313

Report of a Working Party sponsored by the Department of Health and Social Security and convened by the Centre for Policy on Ageing under the Chairmanship of Kina, Lady Avebury.

First published 1984 by the
Centre for Policy on Ageing
Nuffield Lodge Studio
Regent's Park
London NW1 4RS

Reprinted 1984

© 1984 Centre for Policy on Ageing

All rights reserved. No part of this publication may be repro-
duced or transmitted, in any form or by any means without
the prior consent of the copyright owner.

ISBN 0 904 139 37 9

Design
Robert Claxton MSIAD   Beverley M Skinner MSIAD

Printed in Great Britain by
Henry Ling Ltd., The Dorset Press,
Dorchester, Dorset, England

Contents

Foreword by the Secretaries of State

The last few years have seen major developments in voluntary and privately run residential care for elderly people and other vulnerable groups. Private and voluntary homes play a very important part in helping people to remain both near their families or in their own communities, and in avoiding unnecessary stays in hospital.

It is essential that proper standards are set and effective arrangements made to ensure that these are maintained. To this end we are bringing into effect during the course of this year a range of measures designed to improve the registration and inspection of residential care homes and nursing homes.

This code is an important part of the package. We endorse it as an excellent guide to good practice and ask local authorities in carrying out their duties in relation to these homes to regard it in the same light as the general guidance that we issue from time to time under our powers in section 7 of the Local Authority Social Services Act 1970. We also commend the code to people in the private and voluntary sector who have the day to day responsibility for ensuring that good practice is observed.

As Lady Avebury has indicated in her Introduction, the Working Party has striven towards the good rather than simply defined the acceptable. This must be right. These establishments are home for people who live in them and the standards of management and care determine the whole quality of their lives.

The new legislation covers a wide range of establishments, and residents have very different needs. It will be for registration authorities individually to ensure that the code is applied positively and sensitively, in a way that makes sense in local circumstances and has regard to the standards achieved in their own homes.

The Working Party took on a formidable task. However, it brought together members with a wide range of experience, and they have produced a document which should command widespread respect. We are grateful to these members for the way in which they have undertaken their task and in particular to Lady Avebury for the leadership she has given as Chairman. Our thanks go too to the Centre for Policy on Ageing which provided the Working Party with a base as well as a great deal of expert support.

Norman Fowler
Secretary of State for Social Services

Nicholas Edwards
Secretary of State for Wales

Working party membership

Chairman	Kina, Lady Avebury formerly Assistant Director of MIND
Vice Chairman	Mr. Malcolm Johnson Senior Fellow, Policy Studies Institute
	Dr. Michael Apter Senior Lecturer, University of Cardiff and proprietor of a residential care home
	Mr. Paul Brearley Deputy Director (Care), Leonard Cheshire Foundation
	Mr. Richard Clough, MBE General Secretary, Social Care Association
	Mr. Jack Hanson, OBE Director, Social Services Department, Dorset County Council
	Mr. Harry Neal Director, Residential Services, MENCAP
	Miss Alison Norman Deputy Director, Centre for Policy on Ageing
	Mr. Bryan Rowe Registration Officer, Social Services Department, Norfolk County Council
	Mrs. Philippa Russell Senior Officer, Voluntary Council for Handicapped Children
	Dr. Thomas Trace District Medical Officer, South East Kent Health Authority
Official Observers	Miss Phyllis Baldock Social Work Service, Department of Health and Social Security (until June 1983)
	Mrs. Sheila Millington Social Work Service, Department of Health and Social Security (from June 1983)
	Mr. Colin Vyvyan Welsh Office
Secretariat	Ms. Deirdre Wynne-Harley Senior Homes Adviser, Centre for Policy on Ageing
	Mrs. Joyce Cooper Personal Assistant to Ms. Wynne-Harley

Chairman's introduction

This Code of Practice is an integral part of the Government's measures to regulate the establishment and conduct of private and voluntary residential care homes under the *Registered Homes Act 1984*. At the time of publication of this Code, the Act is before Parliament and will become law in late 1984. Under this legislation, the Department of Health and Social Security (DHSS), the Welsh Office and local authorities have powers of inspection of private and voluntary residential care homes. The Code applies to all residential care homes including homes for children registered under the *Registered Homes Act 1984*, but not children's homes registered under the *Child Care Act 1980* or the *Children's Homes Act 1982*. The Working Party which was appointed to produce the Code of Practice has maintained close working contact with the DHSS and with the Welsh Office, and the Code's contents, therefore, relate to, and enlarge upon, the contents of the Act, the Regulations, and the Departmental Memorandum of Guidance to registration authorities. Every effort has been made to ensure that the Code is consistent with legislative requirements and with guidance issued by central government departments. If in any particular instance there should be any inconsistency, the latter should be regarded as prevailing.

At the request of DHSS, the Centre for Policy on Ageing accepted responsibility for both the appointment of the Working Party and for the professional and administrative support which it received. The Centre for Policy on Ageing has an established record in policy analysis and considerable experience in residential care gained through its 'Homes Advice' service to non-statutory residential care homes. The Centre's advisory and technical support preoccupied the working time of several members of the staff for the whole period of the Code's production. In addition the expertise of others was drawn upon freely and with great benefit.

The two principal challenges which have faced the Working Party have been firstly, the wide range of establishments and clients covered by the legislation, and secondly, the need to address more than one audience in the same document.

The legislation encompasses large homes, some of which may be part of a chain of commercial enterprises with home ownership at several removes from management, as well as small family-run homes with as few as four residents. It covers the voluntary and charitable sector as well as the commercial sector. It includes homes providing specialist care for a wide variety of specific client groups, with a wide range of aims and practice, as well as homes run in a more

9

generalist way. The legislation also covers those residential homes which provide nursing care at a level which makes it necessary for them to be registered with their district health authority as well as with the local authority. The residents of all these homes have varying needs. Some of them are in a position to exercise a free choice about where and how to live, whilst others have little or no choice. The extent of their vulnerability, be it physical, psychological or economic, also varies, both between groups and at different periods of an individual's life, and calls for differing patterns of care. The Working Party's concern, in drawing up the Code of Practice, has been to ensure that the care provided in a home accurately reflects the stated aims and objectives of that home, and that it satisfactorily responds to the needs of the residents.

The Code of Practice is intended to assist registration authorities in carrying out their duties of approving and inspecting homes for registration purposes, and to help registration authorities in their advisory and enabling role in relation to proprietors and managers of homes. Equally important, the Code is intended to give direct help to proprietors and managers. The Working Party also hopes that it will be read by the relevant professional workers and members of health and social service authorities, and by all the voluntary bodies concerned with residential care. The wider the circulation the Code receives, the more likelihood there will be of creating a sense of partnership between those responsible for providing the care in homes and those who have a duty to see that high standards of good practice prevail.

Quality of life, as well as quality of care in the strictest sense, is shaped to a very large extent by the attitudes of owners, managers and staff at all levels. For this reason, the Code of Practice attaches considerable weight to the underlying philosophy of care, and to the tenets which give substance to the philosophy. Concepts such as privacy, autonomy, individuality, esteem, choice and responsible risk-taking, provide the foundations and reference points for good practice, and observance of these concepts in all possible circumstances is in itself good practice.

The Code is based upon the belief of all members of the Working Party that there are sufficient common elements of good care, as well as sufficient shared needs and rights of residents, to render too great an emphasis upon particular client groups unnecessary and undesirable. The danger of labelling homes, or the people who live in them, by a single characteristic or disability is that it masks the wider value of residents as people with the same needs and rights as those who do not happen to be living in residential care homes. We recognise, however, that some client groups do have additional special needs, and that there are specific legal obligations to be observed in some cases, so the Code of Practice does offer guidance and information where it is felt to be necessary. Homes which offer care to mentally ill or mentally handicapped people, to children, frail elderly people and to those receiving treatment for alcohol or drug abuse are such instances.

The Working Party has deliberately avoided a detailed prescriptive approach, in the knowledge that what might constitute appropriate levels of care in one home would be unnecessary or unworkable in another. We hope that registration authorities will therefore compare actual practice in a home with its agreed stated purpose, and will feel able, when the need arises, to refer owners and managers to the recognised agencies for further guidance on specialist care. The Code is therefore not a manual or handbook.

The Working Party is aware, in particular, that there are passages in the Code, and specific recommendations, which cannot apply in the case of children in residential care, especially schools. It has borne in mind the fact that children constitute a small minority of people who live in homes, and believes that it will be clear to those concerned which recommendations are inapplicable or unrealistic in such cases. Where homes need dual registration because of the levels of nursing care provided, additional statutory requirements may be enforceable. The registration officer will refer home owners to the relevant departmental Circulars of Guidance. Nevertheless the broad philosophy of the Code is intended to apply universally.

At all times the Working Party has adhered to the aim of fostering good practice, rather than simply delineating the lowest common denominator of minimum standards. The Code of Practice's usefulness is inextricably bound up with the effectiveness of the registration authorities. This, in turn, demands a high degree of commitment on the part of the authorities to provide sufficient experienced and knowledgeable people to undertake the statutory duties in the registration process, and to provide a trusted and accessible resource to those who run the homes in the area. The predicted growth of private and voluntary sector care can be viewed from different perspectives, but there is universal agreement on the need for proper accountability and the monitoring of standards of care. The Working Party's view is that there is nothing in the Code of Practice which should not also apply to the setting up and running of homes in the statutory sector.

The Working Party received a great deal of written evidence, and oral evidence was also given by a number of organisations representing statutory, private and voluntary interests. Its members are grateful to all those organisations and individuals who gave evidence. Many of the proposals have found their way into the Code.

We owe a special debt of thanks to the Centre for Policy on Ageing and to Deirdre Wynne-Harley, its Senior Homes Adviser, in particular. It was she, with the able secretarial support of Joyce Cooper, who organised and administered the programme of work as well as contributing her unrivalled knowledge of the field. Our thanks are also offered to the three observers from central government who have helped us maintain close touch with their colleagues in DHSS and the Welsh Office during the process of legislation, and who have guided us on legal and procedural matters. As Chairman, my own thanks go especially to my fellow members of the Working Party, for sharing their particular skills and experience, and for so readily giving time, individually and collectively, to produce this Code of Practice. Their support at all times has been greatly valued.

Kina Avebury,
Chairman, Code of Practice Working Party

Glossary of definitions

Wherever possible definitions used in this Code are taken from the *Registered Homes Act 1984* and the Regulations governing the conduct of registered homes. For clarification however, certain other terms are also defined below for purposes of this Code.

Residential care home: '.... any establishment which provides or is intended to provide, whether for reward or not, residential accommodation with both board and personal care for four or more persons in need of personal care by reason of old age, disablement, past or present dependence on alcohol or drugs or past or present mental disorder'. (*Registered Homes Act 1984*).

Personal care means care which includes assistance with bodily functions where such assistance is required.

The **responsible person-in-charge** is the person responsible for the day-to-day management of the care of residents.

The **manager** may be the responsible person-in-charge of day-to-day care, or may be concerned solely with business or financial affairs of the home.

'Responsible person-in-charge' or 'the manager' applies equally to private and voluntary homes.

Proprietor indicates ownership of a private establishment and does not mean the appointed manager of a private establishment.

Sometimes the proprietor is also the 'manager'. In a voluntary home the term 'proprietor' relates to the governing body or management committee.

Registration authority is the local authority with responsibility for social services in the area in which the home is situated.

Dual registration refers to homes which are registered both with the registration authority and the health authority.

'He' should in all cases be taken to include 'she'.

1   Principles of care

1.1   Introduction

Underlying all the recommendations and requirements set out in this Code is a conviction that those who live in residential care should do so with dignity; that they should have the respect of those who support them; should live with no reduction of their rights as citizens (except where the law so prescribes), and should be entitled to live as full and active a life as their physical and mental condition will allow.

Whether young or old, sound in mind and body or suffering from disability, residents have a fundamental right to self-determination and individuality. Equally, they have the right to live in a manner and in circumstances which correspond, as far as is possible, with what is normal for those who remain in their own homes.

1.2   The rights of residents

These basic rights should be accorded to all who find themselves in the care of others. In elaborating such rights below, there has been no attempt to distinguish between the requirements of one group of residents and another. Yet it must be recognised that all cannot apply equally to every resident, regardless of his or her condition. Where there are necessary variations, they are indicated in later sections of the Code.

1.2.1 Fulfilment

The purpose of a home should be to enable residents to achieve their potential capacity — physical, intellectual, emotional and social. This can best be achieved by sensitive recognition and nurturing of that potential in each individual and by an understanding that it may change over time.

1.2.2 Dignity

The preservation of self respect amongst those who depend on the support of others hinges upon the status they are accorded. Privacy of space is important as is the right to hold and express opinions or to keep them private. Recognition of talents, sensitivities and beliefs should be an essential feature of the way staff respond to residents. So, too, should courtesy and respect in all relationships; in particular, a respect for what is personal and private.

1.2.3 Autonomy

Living in a community with others requires that residents should recognise and respond to the rhythms and needs of other people. Within these limitations, however, residents have a basic right to self-determination, and they should not, for example, be regimented or subjected to rigid routines.

Within these same limitations, the provision of choice is

an essential principle. The exercise of choice requires a partnership between residents and staff, in which choices can be negotiated and agreed. Some residents — many of them very vulnerable people — will need help to express their wishes and preferences. All residents should have access to external advice, representation and, possibly, advocacy. Even deeply held views and aspirations may not be expressed if staff do not encourage such links outside the home.

1.2.4 Individuality

Staff should be responsive to the needs and requirements of individual residents and not merely impose regimes which are dictated by the needs and preferences of others. For example, the number of residents from ethnic minority communities who come into residential care homes will increase. Staff should be aware of, and provide for, religious, ethnic and cultural observances, both dietary and ritual. Residents with different ethnic backgrounds should be able to feel that their needs will be responded to willingly by staff who understand the value of maintaining the sense of continuity and identity based on past traditions and practices. All residents should be allowed reasonable idiosyncrasy in matters such as dress, food preferences, bed-times and the general run of daily activities.

As well as providing an environment which nurtures individuality and self-awareness, staff of homes should build up, in those who are capable, the self-confidence and motivation to leave for a more independent form of living. Not all residents have a permanent need for residential care, but some may become conditioned into comfortable dependence. When it is in their best interest, individuals should be encouraged to move into more appropriate settings, possibly with a degree of continuing support.

Provision for leisure activities, in and outside the home, is essential. This should be sensitive to individual tastes and capacities and flexible enough to match them. Resources existing in the neighbourhood should be engaged to help meet the needs of residents.

1.2.5 Esteem

It is easy to under-estimate the qualities, experiences and talents of people in residential care and in so doing to lower their morale.

A knowledge of and respect for the individual's life history creates identity for both residents and staff. A positive regard for family and friends, where they exist, reinforces the esteem in which residents are held. It may be helpful for residents to have some knowledge of the life experience of staff, to act as a bridge between them. This emphasises personal connections outside the home and their relevance to those within.

16

1.2.6 Quality of experience

The quality of life in a home will be enhanced by inclusion of the widest possible range of normal activities, particularly those with which residents have been familiar in the past. The presence of personal possessions is extremely important, as are continuing opportunities to go shopping, attend places of worship, visit the cinema, theatre, pubs, clubs, discos and the like. Opportunities should be made available for religious and political beliefs to be expressed and pursued. This may involve recognition of practices such as prayer and contemplation which require privacy and quietness.

1.2.7 Emotional needs

Residents should have normal opportunities for emotional expression, in particular the freedom to have intimate and personal relations within, and outside, the home.

There are, of course, some risks in close relationships and sexual liaisons, especially for young people. These risks may be linked to exploitation or particular instances of emotional vulnerability. General rules which totally ban sexual relations within the home or which allow total permissiveness are undesirable. Individuals will vary in their ability to form and cope with any relationship. Where doubt exists, appropriate specialist consultation should be sought (perhaps via the registration authority) and counselling for the individuals concerned may be considered.

The ability to manage relationships and to assume personal responsibility will also fluctuate over time. Nonetheless, residents will continue to have the same needs as other people for expressive behaviour and physical human contact and these needs should be respected.

1.2.8 Risk and choice

Responsible risk-taking should be regarded as normal, and residents should not be discouraged from undertaking certain activities solely on the grounds that there is an element of risk. Excessive paternalism and concern with safety may lead to infringements of personal rights. Those who are competent to judge the risk to themselves should be free to make their own decisions so long as they do not threaten the safety of others.

2   Social care

2.1

Admission procedures

2.1.1 Introductory brochure

All homes should make available a brochure or prospectus which sets out the aims and objectives of the management, including the type of resident catered for, the degree of care offered, the extent to which illness or disability can be accommodated and any restrictions relating to age, sex, religion etc. The brochure should also accurately describe the facilities, staffing and accommodation offered and may include terms and conditions (see 2.2).

While limited home nursing care may be made available to residents, and reference to this made in the brochure, proprietors must not imply that the establishment is a nursing home. If in doubt, reference should be made to the registration authority as to what statement is permissible and to ascertain whether dual registration is required.

2.1.2 Introductory visits

Prospective long-term residents should visit the home, so that an informed personal decision relating to the application for admission can be made. Similarly, it is also desirable that the proprietor or his representative should visit the prospective resident at his present accommodation so as to establish a personal relationship, gain information about his way of life and advise on possessions which can be accommodated in his room. This will, of course, depend on such a visit being acceptable to the resident. There will be many instances when a social worker could facilitate such introductions.

2.1.3 Short-stay care

Short-stay care is often necessary in an emergency, and may be beneficial on a regular basis. However regard should be paid to the potentially disruptive effect this can have on the home. Wherever possible the need for short-stay accommodation should be met by the provision of separate units. When this is not possible, care should be taken to ensure that the balance of life in the home is not disturbed unduly by the presence of short-stay residents.

2.1.4 Trial stay

The first two months, or longer, after a resident enters a home on a long-term basis should be mutually recognised as a trial period. This allows time to see how well the new resident fits in and allows the resident to change his mind. It is therefore advisable for proprietors to ensure that alternative arrangements will be made for residents if the placement proves unsuitable. Caring relatives or others concerned with their welfare should be made aware of the nature of the trial period. Similarly, adult residents coming from their own homes should be warned not to take any irrevocable step, such as selling a house or terminating a tenancy, until they are certain that they want to stay. Before admission a full physical and, if appropriate, psychological or educational assessment is a sensible requirement.

2.1.5 Review of placement

After the trial period the proprietor should discuss fully with the prospective resident and key supporter (relative, friend, social worker) the suitability of the placement and the prospective resident's feelings about it. The possibility of transfer, if the placement is unsuitable, and eventual discharge, should also be raised if appropriate. Review decisions should be recorded and implemented.

2.1.6 General reviews

On admission a programme of general reviews should be established and the purpose and process of the reviews explained. These reviews will include general health and social needs, and should always be regarded as an opportunity to extend methods of rehabilitation and prepare residents for leaving when this is appropriate. The resident and key supporter should normally be amongst those involved in such reviews. In the case of children in the care of a local authority, reviews are a statutory obligation.

2.1.7 Personal possessions

Residents should be encouraged to bring with them as many personal possessions as can be accommodated in their rooms and close co-operation should be offered in helping the resident to select such items. All residents' possessions should be treated with care and respect, and any valuable items noted. Unobtrusive procedures for the recording of major additions and deletions should be established. Care should always be taken to safeguard personal belongings such as dentures, spectacles and hearing aids.

2.1.8 Personal clothing

It may be necessary for staff to assist a resident with the purchase of new clothes. The practice of supplying clothes from a communal pool is never acceptable.

2.2 Terms and conditions of residence

2.2.1 Written statement of terms and conditions

Before applying for admission, the resident, and where necessary his sponsor, should be given in writing a clear statement of the terms under which the accommodation is offered. This may be included in the introductory brochure if the proprietor so wishes. (See 2.1.1. above.) The statement should include:

- The level of fees, time and method of payment, whether in advance or arrears.
- The services covered by fees.
- Extra services which are charged separately (these should not include any essential facilities).
- Procedure for increasing fees when this is necessary (increases should not normally exceed the prevailing rate of inflation).

19

- The personal items which the resident will be expected to provide for himself.
- Information regarding the home's policy on pets.
- The terms under which the resident can vacate his accommodation temporarily.
- The circumstances in which the resident might be asked to leave.
- Procedure on either side for terminating the agreement or giving notice of changes.
- Statement of insurance of the home and responsibility for insuring personal valuables (amounts of cover for residents' property should be made clear and details of insurers given).
- A statement to the effect that the home is registered as a residential care home by the local authority which is responsible for seeing that standards are maintained.
- A statement to the effect that the home is not registered as a nursing home by the health authority unless dual registration is in force, in which case the situation should be explained.
- Procedure for making complaints to the proprietor and information on how to contact the registration authority in the case of unresolved complaints.
- Procedure on the death of a resident (this should take account of the known wishes of the resident and his social and cultural traditions).

2.2.2 Health

It should be recognised that the person in charge of the home needs to be informed of factors which may affect the type of care required. These will include the prospective resident's medical condition and prognosis together with any relevant social circumstances. Such information will of course be obtained with the consent of the resident (if he is competent) and treated in the strictest confidence.

2.3   **General administration**

2.3.1 Records

Certain records concerning personal details of residents and other matters, are required to be kept under various Regulations. These are referred to in Annexe 3, Model 2. Such records must be open to inspection by the registration authority on request. Personal details in these records must be kept in a secure place and access should be limited to those with overall responsibility for the day-to-day care of the resident. Anyone who has access to records should be instructed in the proper handling of confidential information. Residents' normal rights of access to their personal records should not be unreasonably denied. Managers and staff should be adequately briefed on issues relating to confidentiality and access to case files.

2.3.2 Domestic routines	Domestic routines are necessary for the smooth running of a home, but they need to take into account both individual needs and preferences and the desirability of a lifestyle which is as normal as possible, especially in relation to bathing, getting up, going to bed and mealtimes. Routines should be applied in a friendly, understanding way and offer maximum possible choice, dignity and privacy to residents.
2.3.3 Rules	Rules relating to residents should be kept to a minimum and employed only to promote rehabilitation (under an agreed contract with the resident), fulfil statutory requirements, prevent undue disturbance to other residents or ensure reasonable standards of safety and hygiene. Proprietors should distinguish between behaviour which endangers or seriously inconveniences others and behaviour which involves only the individual concerned. The latter, such as bathing unassisted or going out unaccompanied, should be restricted only if the resident is not capable of making an informed decision on his own responsibility, or if it runs counter to an existing contractual therapeutic regime.
2.3.4 Resident involvement in decision-making	Residents should be involved as much as possible in making decisions concerning the way in which a home is run. Decisions about areas for non-smokers will be important to many people. Menu planning and choice of food, including ethnic and religious options where appropriate, should involve residents. In particular, social or other activities should not be forced upon residents and should not be introduced without consultation. Involvement will, however, depend on the ability and interest of residents and may be as suitably done informally, as by way of formal residents' meetings. Residents or their representatives should have reasonable access to the proprietor or management committee, or their responsible representative, to express their views when they wish to do so.
2.3.5 Modes of address	It is important to take account of individual preference in the way names are used. A person is entitled to be called what he or she wishes, whether it be Mrs. Brown, Alice Brown or Alice. Names are not only labels of identity, they are personal possessions to be handled in the manner their owners choose. Moreover, it is reasonable to wish to be addressed in different ways by different people. Even when an adult invites his fellow residents and, say, the head of home to use his first name, he may still prefer domestic staff and any strangers to call him Mr.
2.3.6 Personal competence	There will be occasions when there is doubt about whether a resident is able or competent to make decisions on his own behalf. This may be as a result of intellectual changes or limitations or some other cause. The law makes provision for certain situations and where any doubt exists about the

competence of any resident, advice should be sought from the registration authority or appropriate independent legal, medical or social work sources.

2.3.7 Complaints procedure

Any infringement of this Code of Practice should normally be considered a legitimate cause for complaint. Other issues not covered in the Code may, of course, arise. All complaints should be treated seriously and recorded. They should never be dismissed automatically as without foundation because of the personal characteristics or mental capacity of the complainant. It follows that a resident should be able to bring complaints on any subject to the proprietor without fear of incurring disapproval, and if he is not satisfied with the outcome, he or someone on his behalf should be able to take the matter up with the registration authority.

2.3.8 Residents' access to personal records

People in residential care should normally be able to discover what is said about them in the personal records maintained by the home. It is good practice for staff to share information with residents in the context of an open, professional relationship. Therefore, subject only to adequate safeguards, residents who wish to have access to written records should be enabled to do so, although in some instances sensitive information may need to be disclosed during special interpretive counselling. In wholly exceptional circumstances certain safeguards will be needed:

- information about a third party should not be disclosed to a resident without the consent of that third party.
- information derived in confidence from a third party should not be disclosed without the consent of the third party.
- information about a child should not be given to parents without the child's permission (unless the child is precluded by age or mental disorder from giving an informed consent).
- in exceptional circumstances it may be concluded after the most careful assessment that, for example, a resident's instability or lack of insight is such that he will need to be protected from the disclosure of matters which have for him a special and damaging significance.
- in wholly exceptional circumstances the longer-term interests of the resident may require the protection of confidential judgements made and recorded by members of staff.

Any decisions to withhold requested information should be taken only at senior level within the organisation responsible for the home; in such a case the resident may appeal to the registration authority and the registered person should be able to explain the reason for the decision to the satisfaction of the registration authority if called upon to do so. The need to withhold access to sensitive items within the record should never be used to justify withholding access to the remainder.

2.4 Residents' security of tenure

The security of tenure enjoyed by any resident will depend on many factors and if there is any doubt about this then it will be the duty of the proprietor to refer the resident to a local Citizens Advice Bureau (CAB) which holds lists of local solicitors, or to the local Law Society, so that the resident can receive independent legal advice. It should be remembered that in most cases residents cannot be evicted from the home without a Court Order.

2.5 Privacy and personal autonomy

2.5.1 Private space

It is highly desirable that all residents in long-term care should have their own room (unless they prefer otherwise), as well as the use of communal areas. Private rooms should be looked after as much as possible by the resident, with staff, in normal circumstances, entering by permission of the resident. Ideally doors should be lockable from both sides, staff members holding a master key. If the rooms in established homes cannot be fully divided to provide private accommodation, every effort should be made to create 'private space' by the use of room dividers and other furniture. Residents should be encouraged to 'personalise' their private space with the use of their own soft-furnishings, ornaments, pictures, plants, etc., and, as far as possible, furniture. Each resident should have the use of an easy chair in his private space, lockable storage and sufficient room for the storage of personal possessions and hanging space for clothing. Residents who so wish should be able to have their own television set. As these rooms should be available for sitting in during the day, they should be kept at a similar temperature to that of the rest of the home. In homes catering for elderly and physically handicapped people, an emergency call system should be installed, though the availability of this should not be used as a means of avoiding appropriate personal contact. All residents should be able to dress, wash and use the toilet in private, even when needing assistance. Residents should be able to meet whom they wish in private, either in their own room or some other comfortable accommodation. Privacy and autonomy should also be promoted by the provision of an appropriately positioned or moveable coin-operated telephone, suitable for use by disabled people, including those who are hard of hearing, if appropriate, and by the opportunity for long-term residents who have their own rooms to install a personal telephone at their own expense.

2.5.2 Activities

Residents should be encouraged to pursue existing interests

or acquire new ones and to help around the home, provided such activities do not interfere unduly with others. Residents who are able to go out alone for walks, shopping and all other social activity should be encouraged to do so. It should be a normal courtesy that if residents go out they should give an indication of their whereabouts and when they will return. If after careful assessment a resident is considered to be too much at risk to go out alone, he should be given as much opportunity as possible to go shopping, for example, with other people. All residents should be enabled to make use of community facilities such as sports centres, hairdressing, chiropody, public library and specialist services. They should also be able to go out freely for trips, meals and longer visits with relatives, friends or volunteers, although they should normally let staff know of their plans. Transport may need to be provided for some of these activities.

Activities both inside and outside the home arising from religious and political beliefs should be respected, provided they do not interfere unduly with others.

It is important that residents be encouraged and enabled to take holidays away from the residential care home. These may be in groups or individually as appropriate, and as the resident wishes. Assistance, information and finance is provided by many voluntary organisations as well as social service departments.

2.5.3 Visitors

Families and friends of residents should be encouraged to visit regularly and maintain contact by letter or telephone when visiting is not possible. Staff may need, in certain circumstances, to offer help to residents in responding. Visitors should be welcomed at all reasonable times, although they should normally let the person in charge know when they come and go. They should also let the person in charge know if the visit has been in any way upsetting. A resident has the right to refuse to see a visitor, and the proprietor should respect this right, accepting responsibility, if necessary, for informing the visitor of the resident's wishes. In occasional instances, a proprietor may have reason to believe that it would be contrary to a resident's best interests to see a particular person. If the proprietor decides to exclude a person from the home, he should record the fact and be able to explain the reasons to the satisfaction of the registration authority if called upon to do so.

2.5.4 Volunteers

Many residents in homes may be without close family ties or friends, possibly because they have had to move some distance from their own homes, or because they have spent some time in other institutions. Volunteers from the surrounding community can do much to lessen this personal sense of isolation, if they are invited and welcomed into a home. There are several ways in which voluntary helpers can assist: by befriending individual residents, by accompanying them to shops, letter writing, inviting them to their own homes, offering themselves as agents to act on behalf of a resident, and dealing with the drawing of benefits. In such instances it would be correct practice for character references to be offered and taken up, and the registration authority provided with the names of volunteers acting in this capacity. One great value of volunteers is the time they can give to listening to and talking with residents, supplementing the staff role in social contact.

2.6 Financial affairs

2.6.1 Wills

Adult residents should be encouraged, tactfully, by their relatives or sponsors, to make a will prior to admission to the home. For those who do not do so, then information about where independent advice and assistance can be obtained should be made available, not only to the resident but, where necessary, to his relatives or sponsors as well. Because it is essential that the advice and assistance given is seen to be independent, it is important that residents are not referred, for instance, to the proprietor's own solicitor. The resident should have a choice, and this can best be achieved by referring him to the local Citizens Advice Bureau which holds lists of local solicitors, or to the local Law Society. Proprietors and staff should not, except in the most extreme emergency, act as witnesses to any resident's will. In no circumstances should the proprietor or any member of the staff become an executor of a resident's will. Where residents clearly have become mentally incapable of making a will, the only body that can do so on behalf of the resident is the Court of Protection (see 2.6.5).

2.6.2 Gifts made in the resident's lifetime

As with wills, the choice about what a resident does with his money is his own. However, because of the close relationship and dependence between the resident and those who manage and run the home, there is a need for a clear statement about the home's attitude to all personal gifts from residents. Ideally, and in order to avoid all suspicion of undue influence, the proprietor should make known to all staff and residents that it is the home's practice to decline all personal gifts, except for small token presents. Tipping of staff should be barred and a note of this, together with the prohibition on receipt of all other gifts, save those referred to above, should be included in each staff member's contract of employment. If, however, a resident is insistent on making a gift, then he must be advised to seek independent advice and ideally the proprietor or member of staff should also seek such advice before deciding what to do.

Discussion with a senior officer of the registration authority would be a satisfactory way of resolving such uncertainty.

2.6.3 Valuables

Residents should be made aware that they are responsible for the safe-keeping of their own money, documents such as pension books, and other valuable possessions, unless some severe mental impairment makes this impossible. The home must have a secure facility, such as a safe or lockable cupboard (with access controlled by the proprietor or manager); and residents should be encouraged to use this and should be given receipts when money or articles are put in it. The home should also keep a permanent register detailing the names of the depositing residents, description of the items deposited for safe-keeping, the date of deposit and subsequent withdrawal. Arrangements for regular withdrawals and deposits may be necessary. Residents should be fully informed about any insurance cover applying to the home which affects their own possessions and, if necessary, should be able to take out their own insurance cover.

If a resident has to be temporarily admitted to hospital or leaves the home for some other purpose, he should be able to leave all valuables in the safe or some other secure place and be given a receipt. In the case of the resident's inability to do this, the agent who acts on his behalf should take responsibility.

2.6.4 Appointment of agents, trustees and attorneys by residents who are legally competent

A resident may nominate a relative, friend or someone in the community over the age of 18 to act as his agent in drawing and making payments. There is a well-established procedure for doing this for social security payments. If the resident wants a third party to operate his bank account then he can instruct a bank accordingly. When there is no relative or friend available whom the resident trusts, the local social services department should be asked to recommend someone to act as his agent. The names of suitable individuals or organisations should be lodged with the registration authority.

The proprietor or manager should not take on this role unless it has proved impossible to find an alternative. The proprietor should notify the social services department of residents for whom this arrangement is made. Such arrangements should be strictly limited to weekly payments only and should not apply to any capital or assets.

If a resident wishes to delegate more extensive powers to act on his behalf, he may execute a power of attorney under which he gives authority to someone else to undertake this role. Such a power may be limited in time or extent at the resident's discretion but it becomes technically invalid if the resident becomes legally incompetent. (If this should happen, any agreement which is made by the attorney with a third party who does not know of the resident's incapacity, remains binding.) Again a solicitor should always be consulted when making a power of attorney and in no circumstances should anyone connected with the management of the home be appointed attorney.

Alternatively, a resident may decide to set up a trust to manage his affairs. This is normally worth doing only if there are substantial assets but it has the great advantage of continuing to be valid even if the resident should cease to be mentally competent.

2.6.5 Management of the affairs of residents who are not legally competent

If a resident is in receipt of social security payments and is assessed by a qualified medical practitioner as being mentally unable to act for himself, his agent (if he has previously nominated someone in this role), relative, or if necessary the manager or proprietor, should immediately notify the local social security office responsible for the payment of that resident's benefit and provide the office with details of a suitable person to act on his behalf, if necessary seeking a social services recommendation (as in 2.6.4 above). Again it is most undesirable that a manager or proprietor should take on this role whatever the pressures.

If a resident has more substantial financial assets, an application should be made to the Court of Protection (Staffordshire House, Store Street, London WC1) for the resident to be placed under the jurisdiction of the Court. Such an application is most appropriately made by a resident's relative, sponsor or social worker but it can be done by anybody. It must be accompanied by a medical certificate indicating the nature of the person's disorder and its effect upon his capacity to manage his own affairs. (The relevant forms are obtainable from the Court together with advice on procedure.) If the application is accepted, the Court may appoint a receiver to manage the resident's affairs and may also, if it is thought necessary, make a will on the resident's behalf. There is a modified procedure which is used when the resident's assets are not extensive enough to justify a receiver. Although proprietors have no legal obligation to defend the interests of residents who are no longer capable of looking after their financial affairs, it is recommended that they should initiate the appropriate action where there is nobody else capable or willing to do so. Prior discussion with the registration authority is essential. If referral to the Court of Protection seems indicated, the appropriate action would be for the proprietor to draw the matter to the attention of the resident's GP and, if he indicates a willingness to provide the necessary medical recommendation, then, in the absence of any other appropriate person, the proprietor should contact the Court of Protection for advice and, if necessary, make the application himself. Under no circumstances should anybody connected with the running of the home be appointed receiver.

2.6.6 Children's financial affairs	The general principles indicated in this section of the Code apply equally to children as to adults. However proprietors do have a professional responsibility for educating children in the management of money.
2.6.7 Conclusion	Those involved in the running of residential homes have no legal obligations to see that the law is complied with where residents' financial affairs are concerned, save where they become involved themselves in some way. However, if they feel that something (not necessarily of a legal nature) is going wrong, and the resident is unable to deal with it himself, proprietors should draw their fears to the attention of the relatives or registration authority, whichever is most appropriate.

This duty in no way contradicts the essential principle that all those connected with the running of a home should *not* become involved in the handling and management of a resident's financial affairs. Proprietors are potentially very vulnerable to accusations of misconduct. |

2.7 Health care

2.7.1 Health services	Admission to a home in no way diminishes a resident's right of access to the health and remedial services available in the community. This includes the right to choose his own general practitioner and to see him in private. Proprietors, with the consent of the resident, should be kept informed of any necessary changes in the resident's care. The rights of residents to have access to community nursing services does not in any way put at risk the registration of the home as a residential care home. (Appropriate guidance is given in the DHSS/ Welsh Office Memorandum *Residential homes for the elderly: arrangements for health care*, DHSS circular HC(77)25, LAC(77)13 and Welsh Office circular 117/ 77, WHC(77)30.) Proprietors have a right of access to available community resources and advice in the interests of their residents.
2.7.2 Consent to treatment	The law provides that no medical treatment can be given to any person without his valid consent. Any breach of this rule will render the person in breach liable to legal proceedings. A number of elements are necessary for consent to be 'valid'; sufficient information should be given to the patient about the proposed treatment; the patient should be competent to consent, and give consent voluntarily. In the case of a resident belonging to an ethnic minority who has difficulty in communicating in English, every effort must be made to find an interpreter who will explain on behalf of the practitioner the purpose and effect of the proposed treatment, and if necessary explain on behalf of the resident any anxieties or objections he may have.

People over the age of 18 can lawfully consent to medical |

treatment. Those between 16 and 18 can also lawfully consent to medical treatment (Family Law Reform Act 1969). Whether children under 16 can lawfully consent will depend on the understanding of the child and the nature of the procedure which it is intended to carry out. Where those under 16 cannot validly consent, parents or those acting *in loco parentis* stand in the child's stead and can consent to treatment for which the benefit to the child outweighs the harm (not *any* treatment). In wardship and care proceedings the Court will act only on someone else's initiative and not on its own, but if the matter is brought to its notice, the Court will decide what is in the best interests of the child.

.7.3 Administration of drugs

No drugs except simple 'household remedies' should be given without a doctor's prescription. Not all residents will be able to retain and administer their own prescribed medication, but it is desirable that those who are deemed to be so able, should be encouraged to do so. In making decisions about medication practices within the home, proprietors have a statutory responsibility to make proper arrangements for safe-keeping, administering and disposing of drugs and medicines. Where residents administer their own drugs, facilities should be provided for the safe-keeping of medication in a personal, lockable drawer or cupboard. Drugs for which the proprietor takes responsibility should be kept in a secure place in individual containers, fully labelled with name and dosage, and administered only by a trained, responsible person authorised by the proprietor. Staff responsibility does not extend to insisting upon or making residents take medication. Failure to take prescribed medication should be reported to the resident's general practitioner. A record of drugs received and administered by the home must be maintained. The proprietor has a responsibility for ensuring that staff are trained in the administration of drugs and should seek advice from the registration authority. Medication must never be used for social control and punishment.

.7.4 When treatment can be given without consent

When a person is thought to be 'incompetent' (unconscious or severely mentally disordered for instance), then the law allows necessary treatment to be given without consent in cases of urgent necessity. This is generally defined as covering treatment required to deal with an immediate life-threatening illness or condition.

There are occasions when residents require treatment which is not related to immediate life-threatening illness, but which might have a short- or long-term effect on their health. In such situations residents are responsible for their own decisions. Where the person concerned cannot understand the nature of an operation and anaesthetic, for example, there is no authority in law for a relative or the responsible local authority to give consent.

When a child is in care but parental rights and duties have not passed to the local authority, the consent of the child's parent or guardian to the use of drugs should be obtained. In the case of an emergency when, in the clinical judgement of a consultant psychiatrist or medical practitioner acting in good faith, immediate treatment is needed to protect the child's life and health, such consent need not be obtained if it is not practicable to do so.

The Mental Health Act 1983 allows certain psychiatric treatments to be given without the patient's consent to certain categories of patients suffering from mental disorder who are compulsorily detained in hospital because of that disorder. These provisions may be relevant in this context only when the resident is detained under the Mental Health Act 1983, and is living in the home on leave from a hospital. In these very rare circumstances, the hospital in which the patient is liable to be detained will advise the home about the patient's legal position and any questions should be addressed to the hospital. Any treatment given in this way has to be given by or under the direction of the patient's responsible medical officer, who will be the hospital consultant in charge of the patient's treatment.

2.7.5 Dying and Death

When a home has stated an intention to 'care until death' appropriate terminal care should be provided wherever practical, and the particular skills required fully understood and agreed by all concerned. The importance of obtaining proper support from the community nursing service, the GP and, if necessary, specialists such as a visiting hospice nurse, cannot be over-emphasised. It gives a great sense of security to residents to know that they will not be sent away to die, unless this is unavoidable or they really want specialist care such as a hospice can provide. Intensive or terminal care should be provided in the resident's own room and not in a 'special care unit' which becomes quickly associated in people's minds with 'the end of the road'.

A further dimension of care arises in meeting the physical and emotional needs of a dying resident and he should be made as comfortable as possible, both in body and mind. It is possible that sometimes this care will be best provided in a hospice or hospital. If the resident is aware that he is dying, he should be given the opportunity to express his wishes concerning terminal care, funeral or cremation arrangements, though it is preferable that this should be done informally at an earlier stage. Contact should be made if requested or known to be acceptable, with an appropriate minister of religion.

Relatives should be informed, and enabled to stay with the resident if they wish to do so. It may be helpful to them to talk about their feelings to members of staff, and staff should be aware of this, and help to give the necessary support. Staff will themselves need support in this work, possibly from outside the home. Staff should be aware of procedures to be followed when death occurs and news of the death should be conveyed to other residents in a dignified and sympathetic way, even though the death may occur away from the home. It may be appropriate to consider any local or cultural customs as well as any known preferences of the deceased person and his family. This may include giving residents an opportunity to see their deceased friend. Particular procedures relating to religious belief or ethnic group practice should be ascertained and carefully observed.

Particular problems may arise after a death in connection with the resident's property. Proprietors should know who would take responsibility for property pending the proving of the will. This information should be obtained at an early stage and included in the resident's personal records and checked at intervals.

2.7.6 **Dual registration (see also 6.10)**

The provision for dual registration is to enable the resident to continue to be cared for, without a break, in the same premises when his medical condition improves or deteriorates. While the levels of care in the two kinds of home can 'shade' together, the fundamental difference is that a nursing home is required to provide nursing care of a kind and to such an extent (in numbers of nurses) as the registering authority considers appropriate (1975 Nursing Homes Act: Section 4). This is not to say, however, that a residential care home, solely because it has a qualified nurse or nurses on its staff, is entitled to be registered as a nursing home. The boundary between the need for residential care and for nursing care, and between 'resident' and 'patient', is rarely clear cut, and the dually registered establishment provides an environment which, in principle, is wholly in the interest of the occupants. It follows that the application of the standards of the two sets of legislation by the two registering authorities should be harmonious.

3   **Physical features**

3.1   Introduction

Registration authorities, in prescribing standards for various client groups, will refer to the appropriate Building Notes or any other guidance published by the DHSS and the Welsh Office (see Annexe 1). In the case of older buildings being adapted, such guidance may need to be interpreted flexibly. Standards in registered housing association shared accommodation, including hostels, are governed by the Housing Corporation's design and contract criteria for shared housing.

3.2   Location

Many residential care homes have been sited inappropriately. Registration authorities, in dealing with all new applications, should therefore ensure that the location and the surrounding environment are suited to the stated aims of the establishment, and at the same time provide a setting which enables the home to blend into the neighbourhood. The accessibility of local facilities, community health services and public transport should be considered fully prior to registration.

3.3   Size

The size of the building and the numbers to be accommodated in it should be considered in the context of the stated aims of the home. Developments in recent years have shown that establishments catering for large numbers are unable to provide the type of care which is indicated in other sections of this Code of Practice. The physical size of the building, therefore, should not be the only determinant of the number of occupants of a home. When considering registration, the local authority should satisfy itself that the proposed number of residents in social groupings, as well as the total establishment, is commensurate with the type of care set down in the stated aims.

3.4   Accommodation and space

The aim of the home should be to provide a homely, non-institutional atmosphere which is suited to the needs of people living in it.

The Regulations require reasonable accommodation and space by day and night including that for social and occupational activities. To some extent what is reasonable will be dictated by the stated purpose of the establishment.

All homes should have communal rooms. Whenever possible, separate rooms for residents to follow their own hobbies or chosen activities, and, where necessary, space for children to do homework, should be provided, in addition to a lounge. Flexible use of communal rooms should always be encouraged. Facilities should be provided for residents to meet in private their financial advisers, social workers, relatives and staff, either in residents' own rooms or in a suitable alternative setting.

In homes intended for the frail and disabled, the registration authority will need to ensure that the building is suitable for the degree of disability to be catered for. For example passages and doorways will need to be wide enough to accommodate persons using walking aids and wheelchairs and where appropriate handrails and/or ramps should be provided.

3.5 Residents' own rooms

The stated purpose of the establishment will dictate how many rooms should have single or double occupancy, and such arrangement must be agreed on registration. However, single rooms would normally be considered preferable to shared rooms. In any case, special reasons will be expected where there are more than two people to a room.

Where bedsitting rooms are provided, residents should be encouraged as far as possible to bring their own furniture. This furniture will remain the property of the resident unless he indicates otherwise. Where it is not possible for residents to bring their own, all furniture, bedding and floor coverings provided should be of a normal, domestic type that provides comfort, as well as space for clothes and other belongings.

Luggage should be stored in a room other than the resident's room to allow maximum use of space and to discourage residents from 'living out of suitcases'.

Whether or not residents' rooms are used as sitting rooms, all rooms should have at least one comfortable armchair, a chest of drawers, separate hanging space for the clothes of each resident occupying the room, and a table for multi-purpose use. There should also be somewhere provided for possessions to be locked away safely.

For adults and older children there should be accessible power and light sockets for the use of small electrical appliances and varied lighting. Adjustable lighting for reading in bed should be provided. Trailing flexes must be avoided. For younger children, power and light sockets must not be easily accessible.

Residents should be allowed a choice of bedding and such bedding should be made of flame- and smoulder-resistant material.

Floors should be covered in non-slip material and carpets should not have frayed edges or raised surfaces at joins.

Residents should be able to have their names on the outside of their doors and, where possible, letter boxes and locks provided. Where appropriate, telephones and televisions in residents' rooms should be permitted and use of wall space for pictures and ornaments should be encouraged.

3.6 Washbasins, baths, showers and toilets

There should be a private wash basin within each bedroom; in shared rooms a screened area should surround wash basins. Privacy should be ensured for personal care normally considered private. The overall ratios of bathrooms and toilets should be not less than the minimum indicated in the appropriate Building Note or guidance. These ratios should exclude toilets and bathrooms for staff use only. Provision of some separate showers designed for seated use provides an element of choice and should be allowed. The siting of toilets is as important as the number provided and this factor should be taken into account in planning.

Bath and shower rooms should be designed to enable residents to achieve the greatest degree of independence and privacy possible, whilst recognising some people's need for regular or occasional assistance.

The stated purpose of the establishment will dictate if extra amenities are required and the registration authority must satisfy itself that client need is met in the facilities provided in toilets and bathrooms. Establishments catering for frail or disabled people should be equipped with at least one sluice suitably sited to avoid carrying soiled items too far.

3.7 Laundry facilities

Laundry facilities should always be separated from the kitchen and food preparation areas of the home. Residents may wish to be able to launder their personal clothing for themselves. If this is the case, or if it is seen to be one way of encouraging independence, space should be provided for washing, drying and ironing. Depending upon the wishes and capabilities of the residents, washing machines and drying machines could be usefully made available for their shared use.

3.8 Diet and food preparation

The style of catering, variety and presentation of food reflect the attitudes of those responsible for the running of the home. Consideration of residents' dietary needs and wishes should be seen as integral to the philosophy of the home in allowing maximum choice and flexibility. It is necessary that staff training includes the social and cultural importance of meals, their content and preparation, in addition to the nutritional needs of the particular client group. Whether meals are served centrally or in small group units, choice of dish and portion size are important, and ready plated meals should be avoided. Special needs of residents with eating difficulties should be met discreetly.

Flexibility in the timing of meals, and facilities, either individually provided or in group rooms, for self-made drinks and snacks are significant factors in normalising life in residential care.

Homes should be prepared to cater for special diets whether these are medically advised, of religious, cultural or philosophical significance, or the result of strong preferences. Residents who cannot eat particular foods for any of these reasons should not be deprived of nutritious, appetising alternatives. In order to cater appropriately, it may be necessary to keep separate utensils and areas of the kitchen for the preparation of certain foods. Proprietors should ascertain on admission if a resident has special dietary needs and take advice from the community dietician or religious advisers how these needs can best be met. In all cases the responsible person in charge should ensure that residents are not misled into eating foods they would not otherwise take.

4 Individual client groups

4.1 Introduction

An essential principle of this Code is that homes should recognise and respond to the needs and potential of individual residents, whatever their degree of disability, their age or their circumstances. Throughout the Code, an attempt has been made to deal with residents' needs, requirements and expectations as though they were held in common. In general terms this is true. Whether residents are old or young, handicapped or able-bodied, there are many matters which are fundamental to all who live under the care of others. It would however be unreasonable to take this conviction too far. Children in school clearly do not have the same freedom of action as adults. Elderly people who are suffering from dementia cannot be allowed to jeopardise the safety of others. People in alcohol- and drug-dependency units are often properly subject to regimes which, at least for a period, suspend some of their right to self-determination, for therapeutic purposes. In recognition of these essential differences, the following sections are devoted to the special circumstances which apply to individual client groups. It should be recognised that these short sections are not intended to be comprehensive and that only the main special circumstances are referred to.

Some of the comments on special needs of particular client groups may appear repetitious, but they are written in the knowledge that such needs, unfortunately, often fail to be met, either because the people concerned may not express or recognise their own needs, or because staff are insufficiently trained or experienced to perceive them.

4.2 Physically disabled people

4.2.1 General principles

Disabled people should have the same opportunities as anyone else to make informed choices and, if they wish, to take risks. This principle should apply even if the consequences of actions may be potentially more serious for a disabled person, or if a disabled person is less able, perhaps because of limited mobility, to avoid some hazards.

Disabled people are often reliant on others for help in meeting intimate personal needs and it is particularly important that care is taken to enable them to preserve autonomy and dignity. They will enter residential homes for a variety of reasons and at a wide range of ages. Whether admission is as a result of, for example, progressively increasing incapacity, or as a temporary respite, or for a period of rehabilitation or relearning, it will be essential to provide every possible opportunity for each individual to realise his own potential to the fullest extent.

| 4.2.2 | Residents with communication difficulties | Difficulties in communication, such as those resulting from hearing loss or other sensory deprivations or speech difficulties, can make life particularly difficult and every effort should be made to ensure a satisfactory means of communication. This will involve provision for material requirements (such as radio aids, door alarms and other electronic aids); the training of staff to ensure proper understanding of communication needs; services to ensure the proper fitting, repair and use of aids; and the support and training of disabled people to overcome communication problems. Those with sensory handicaps frequently have difficulty in gaining access to information both of a general and of a personal nature. Staff need to be aware of the nature and extent of these difficulties for each individual and to be able to take steps to alleviate the problem in a practical and sensitive way. |

| 4.2.3 | Special provisions | In all homes it will be necessary to provide: |

- Helpers to assist the resident to carry out those personal and intimate tasks he would do for himself were it not for his disability.
- Specially designed or adapted accommodation to reduce or remove the effects of the disability, in order to maximise independence compatible with motivation and ability.
- Appliances and aids to enable the disabled person to do things which he could not otherwise manage and also to ease the work of helpers. Assistance may be necessary, for instance in the case of children and newly disabled people, to ensure that aids are used to the best advantage.
- Efficient lighting, without glare, is necessary where visually handicapped people are accommodated. To make best use of residual vision, colour contrast to identify doors and furnishings is helpful, as are tactile clues (i.e. raised numbers on doors) to help locate rooms.

| 4.2.4 | Consulting the resident | In making such provisions, it should be remembered that the disabled person himself has the greatest experience of his own needs and disabilities and will usually be the best person to give advice and teaching about the management of his disabilities. Assumptions should not be made without seeking his advice. Even people who have been disabled for a long time may be able to respond positively to a changed environment and the opportunity to learn new skills and techniques and so improve independence. The occupational therapists who are employed by the health authority or social services department can contribute significantly to this process. |

4.3 Mentally ill people and their rehabilitation

| 4.3.1 | Introduction | In the past twenty-five years the number of people discharged from mental illness hospitals into private and |

voluntary homes has risen sharply. The homes that admit people with a history of mental illness vary considerably in their aims and practice. The needs of such residents are also varied and, historically, insufficient care has been taken to ensure that their needs are appropriately met, or that managers of homes receive enough advice and support from discharging hospitals or the local authority responsible for the resident's well-being. Homes which provide such a service range from hotels and boarding houses employing untrained staff to specialist hostels with clearly set out aims and staff who are qualified and experienced in the field of mental illness.

The phrase 'psychiatric rehabilitation hostel' is used to cover a wide variety of establishments. It includes accommodation specifically for people recently discharged from long-stay hospital wards; people who because of histories of personality disorders are unable to live independently; and people who are recovering from acute mental illness and neurotic disorder. A considerable number of residents who leave hospital are no longer mentally ill, but will have acquired the marks of institutionalisation through years spent in hospital. As a result they may be isolated and withdrawn in appearance, passive in behaviour, and find it hard to exercise choice or make friends.

4.3.2 Advice and support to staff

Running accommodation for former psychiatric patients is a highly skilled and demanding task. The registration authority should take particular care to satisfy itself that the home will be run by staff who are qualified or sufficiently experienced to care for the proposed client group, and who have proper advice and support from recognised professionals in the relevant field. Particular caution should be exercised if the proposed regime is outside recognised techniques of care and rehabilitation.

4.3.3 Assessment procedures

The registration authority should also be satisfied that the proposed assessment procedures are likely to ensure that the home does not admit residents for whom, by the nature or degree of their disability, the home is unsuitable or beyond the capabilities of its staff. The home should record the client's legal status under the Mental Health Act 1983, on admission, and note any changes of status which may follow.

4.3.4 Curtailing residents' freedom

Some hostels may limit autonomy and privacy in the interests of rehabilitation. For example, residents may be expected to conform to a strict timetable; share experiences at group meetings; accept group criticism and comment on their behaviour; and surrender their medication. Such a regime, though apparently authoritarian, does recognise the resident's basic autonomy if he has accepted it in a fully-explained and agreed contract.

4.3.5 Encouraging independence Other hostels may accommodate former long-stay psychiatric patients who need help and encouragement to make use of opportunities for autonomy and privacy and require a gentle introduction to self-determination as part of the process of building up their self-esteem. Such residents are likely to progress to independent living at varying speeds and for some the need to cling on to institutional habits may have to be recognised and accepted. Such residents have a particular need to be involved in positive daytime activity and to have the use of neighbourhood resources. The registration authority should satisfy itself that this need will be met. In addition to ensuring that the level of community care is adequate and is available to residents, the authority should consider the active involvement of voluntary agencies, particularly those whose prime concern is with this client group. The disablement resettlement officers at the local Department of Employment can also be approached about any suitable sheltered employment. There is little advantage in leaving a psychiatric hospital where there is a planned programme of activity for a hostel or home in which residents simply vegetate.

4.3.6 Health care If homes admit residents who may still need some treatment from a hospital outside their own health district, they should seek to obtain an undertaking in writing that the hospital will continue to accept responsibility for any continuing or developing psychiatric problems, or that the hospital will, if necessary, arrange for suitable treatment and care to be given locally. The registration authority should satisfy itself that those responsible for discharging patients into their area maintain their after-care and social work responsibilities, or make formal arrangements to pass these responsibilities on to the local authority social services department. If continuing medication is required there should be consultation as to whether the resident should be encouraged to administer it himself. When medication is given at intervals by means of a 'depot' injection (a long-lasting means of stabilising certain conditions), this should be done at the GP's surgery or at a clinic, whichever is most suitable and in accordance with the resident's wishes. Only in exceptional circumstances should it be practice to administer injections in the home or hostel, as this can reinforce the atmosphere of an institution.

The onset of physical illness or infirmity in a former psychiatric patient must be the concern of the local medical services and should not be considered the responsibility of the discharging psychiatric hospital.

In addition, all such hostels and homes are entitled to help from relevant community services provided by either the health authority or social services department, including those provided by community psychiatric nurses, psychologists, day centre managers and occupational therapists.

4.4 Mentally handicapped people

4.4.1 General principles

The objective of any residential home for mentally handicapped people, children and adults, should be to provide a normal living environment in which sustained encouragement, instruction, and stimulation are continuing elements in the daily life of the residents. Although mental handicap is a condition for which there is no cure, there is, at the same time, a potential for learning and development which is too often ignored or under-valued. If mentally handicapped people are to achieve these levels of development, they have to be encouraged to live as normal a life as possible. This may involve taking part in some activities which carry elements of risk. Caring for mentally handicapped people requires a balance between guidance and encouragement to make choices and learn new skills, and support which acknowledges the different degrees of handicap without being unnecessarily protective. The involvement of community psychiatric nurses specialising in mental handicap, and psychologists, can be very helpful in achieving this balance.

4.4.2 Admission, assessment and reviews

The decision to enter into residential care is a matter for the adult concerned, his parents or nearest relatives, together with the supervisory staff who will care for him. Relevant professionals, such as local authority social workers who are already involved in the resident's past care, should also participate. It should be appreciated that clashes between family and professionals sometimes occur and in this situation, the interests and preferences of the client are paramount.

In the case of a child with a statement of special educational needs, the decision to enter into residential care may be the result of the local education authority's (LEA) assessment of needs. The interests of the client may be paramount but not necessarily his preferences. The statement will specify the special educational provision to be made and it will be the duty of the LEA to provide it.

A full assessment of educational and social potential, and of physical and emotional needs of each entrant, is important for residential placement. This should be made or be available prior to or immediately after placement.

Each resident's development should be regularly assessed and recorded. Planned programmes of activities should be implemented by staff with the appropriate skills.

All discussions on progress and any decision making should involve staff, parents or relatives, and the resident.

4.4.3 Social work support

It is essential that every mentally handicapped resident has access to a local authority social worker, or other suitable person able to provide the necessary personal support. If the resident does not already have a social worker assigned to him, proprietors and managers should make arrangements with their local social services office, on the resident's behalf.

4.4.4 Activities, education and training

It is not enough to think of residential care simply in terms of the provision of bed, board and assistance in bodily functions, even for those who appear most able. Appropriate day-time occupation, and full-time education in the case of a child, is of the utmost importance for all mentally handicapped people. In most instances this would mean attendance at a local authority day centre, school, or training unit. Opportunities for open or sheltered employment should be explored, and consideration of this possibility should be one element in the review procedure.

If the resident is not receiving any day care prior to admission, appropriate provision should be sought at the earliest opportunity. The social services department will be able to tell proprietors what resources are available and will assist in making appropriate referrals to statutory or voluntary services. In the case of children, if suitable full-time education is not being provided then referral will be made to the local education authority. If there is no day-care provision, proprietors should indicate in their statement how day-time developmental activities and social stimulus will be provided. However, registration authorities should be careful not to encourage the establishment of homes for mentally handicapped people in areas which have few community resources.

4.4.5 General welfare

Some mentally handicapped people will not be able to plan ahead or secure or provide for themselves those goods and services for which others would be expected to make their own arrangements. Proprietors should accept responsibility for the general welfare of their residents. Part of this responsibility lies in helping to develop independence over a period of time.

Wherever possible residents should be involved in the running of the home in order to experience 'learning through doing'. Supervision is needed to help residents acquire independent living skills, and the fact that work in the home is undertaken by residents should not be taken to mean that fewer staff are needed.

Residents should be encouraged and helped to take holidays individually or in small groups, as provided for in the Chronically Sick and Disabled Persons Act 1970. Social services departments will advise on the many national and local voluntary agencies who may help fund holiday costs.

Professional specialist workers should be available to advise and support the staff of the home and to give any necessary care or treatment to residents.

Arrangements for dental examinations, eyesight tests and hearing tests, if appropriate, should be made every six months.

4.5 Children and young people

4.5.1 Introduction

Most of the guidance in this Code applicable to the care of adult residents applies also in relation to children. There are however emotional, psychological and developmental factors which are particular to child residents and which require different responses.

Children in homes cannot be viewed in isolation from their feelings about absent parents and their own family settings. Their ability to function at all will be governed by the awareness of care staff of the importance of these background factors, the divided loyalties between parent and care staff this might cause in a child's mind, and the feelings of guilt which the child might retain as being the cause of any family difficulties or breakdowns. Young children and adolescents will exhibit their feelings in different ways and by different behaviour, and care staff should respond, not to any hostile symptoms, but to the anxieties which underlie these.

The interests of child residents are protected by laws which do not apply to adults and care staff should be made aware by the responsible social worker of the way any such laws may affect treatment of the child. Staff should also be fully informed of any provisions made by an order of the Court or constraints imposed by common law.

4.5.2 General principles

The quality of personal relationships between a child and care staff is of the utmost importance. Thus, the staff should have some awareness, on the one hand, of attachment behaviour by young children to a consistent, caring adult, and the expectations a young child might consequently have of individual members of staff. On the other hand, because the element of control is more crucial, especially with adolescents, so also is the need to achieve co-operation rather than confrontation.

Care staff need to recognise that children coming into residential care will be anxious and will want to feel accepted although their behaviour may disguise this fact. As anxiety can produce anger and aggressive behaviour, the carers should understand these reactions and respond appropriately to the needs of a distressed and unhappy child. Although staff are not to be seen as substitute parents in a narrow sense of the word, they should endeavour to provide a warm and caring environment, which fosters and develops good personal relationships between staff and children at all times and which meets children's needs for security, reassurance of personal worth, stimulation and affection.

Children have to be helped to understand their need to be in residence and the reality of their situation. This should be done by repeated explanations in as many ways as possible, otherwise a child may merely see his carers as stopping him from going home.

The general needs of children make it undesirable that they should be accommodated in homes caring for elderly or very ill people.

4.5.3 Planning goals

Goal planning for the child and regular reviewing of this development, involving the child wherever possible, is crucial. The planning should cover long-term matters taking into account the entire period the child will be in the establishment, as well as achievable short-term objectives. The plans made should not make unrealistic demands on the child. They should reflect a child-centred philosophy which provides maximum opportunity for each child to mature and develop as an individual and to express choice and accept responsibility. Children of both sexes need opportunities to develop daily living skills, such as handling money, shopping, cooking and simple repairs.

The accurate recording of past events in a child's life, the retaining of photographs and the compilation of a 'life story book' may be of major importance.

4.5.4 Controls and sanctions

Controls and sanctions should not be applied in such a manner as to undermine the self-respect of children or to lessen their sense of responsibility. Where possible, intervention should be based on reward rather than punishment, with the emphasis placed on good relationships and honesty, trust and respect. However, where sanctions have to be introduced, these should have as their objective the growth of self-discipline otherwise they become merely repetitive. Early bedtime, the setting of additional tasks, the restriction of entertainments and the temporary withholding of pocket money are preferable to other measures which might humiliate the child in the eyes of himself and his peers. Restricting a child's contact with his parents or depriving him of food should not be used as forms of correction, nor should restriction of liberty be used.

Behaviour modification, a recognised form of treatment used in some psychiatric hospitals and to a certain extent in residential care, should only be undertaken on the instruction of a medical practitioner or psychologist and under strict supervision. It should not be practised loosely by untrained workers as a means of discipline. (See Annexe 4; Behaviour Modification).

Corrective measures which are taken must be recorded and the records must be available for inspection by authorised persons. A clear and written policy about sanctions should be understood by staff, and its execution closely super-vised by the head of the home. Medication must never be administered for purposes of social control or punishment.

4.5.5 Relation-ships with parents

The importance of absent parental figures to a child should be recognised and the extent to which parents can share and be responsible for decisions affecting the child should be maximised. If there is no family contact, it is essential that the child be helped to feel safe to talk about his parents with understanding adults and be helped with his divided loyalties towards care staff and his parents.

When parents do visit the establishment, they in turn might feel guilty and inadequate because someone else is caring for their child. They might react by being critical of the carers or by being over-anxious or by failing to visit as promised. Care staff might find it difficult in these circum-stances to have a dispassionate and non-critical attitude towards parents, but carers who can understand the natural parents' feelings and can offer reassurance will be helping to increase the child's own confidence.

4.5.6 Handi-capped children

Caring for children with an identified mental or physical handicap requires an additional range of staff knowledge. Such youngsters are likely to require the support of a specialist network of local services from outside the estab-lishment, and care staff will need factual knowledge about the sources of such help locally and the manner in which it is enlisted. Carers should however also recognise that handicapped children have more in common with other chil-dren than is often assumed. The need for emotional security is as great for these children as for any other child. Some-times staff have a low expectation of handicapped children and a belief in the need for excessive control and authority, but they cannot be cocooned from any risk if they are to develop their full potential and their wishes should be taken into account as with all residents.

4.5.7 Legal status of children

The legal position of a child should be clearly identified at the outset. The staff of the establishment should obtain information about which decisions can legally be made by the child or by the staff, and which decisions require refer-ence to others (for example a local authority if the child is in care), which parent has legal custody, whether a guardian has been appointed, or whether the child is a ward of court.

4.5.8 The education authority

Handicapped children are entitled to education under the provisions of the Education Act 1981 and proprietors must make every effort to ensure that appropriate educational provision is made available for *all* children in their care. As the Education Act 1981 requires local education authorities (LEAs) to assess and make statements of the special edu-cational needs of all children who have severe or complex disabilities or learning difficulties, discussions prior to placement should include contact with both the LEA of the child's place of origin and with the LEA within which the residential home is located. Full assessment under the new procedures will provide detailed information on a child's abilities as well as his deficits, and on strategies for meeting any special needs. Indeed, it will usually be this assessment of a child's needs which leads to a residential placement. The statement will specify the special educational provision to be made and it will be the duty of the LEA to provide it, or to be satisfied that suitable arrangements are being made by the child's parents. In producing the statement, the LEA should take full account of the parents' views, as well as professional advice; the feelings of the child should also be considered.

Wherever possible, handicapped children should attend a local day school. The care staff will benefit greatly from discussions with the teachers in that school, as well as with contacts with the school health and psychological services which, in this instance, can provide a method of monitoring the child's development as well as advising on specific health or behavioural problems.

In certain circumstances, handicapped children may be placed in registered residential homes which provide education on the premises. In these instances, the child's emotional and social needs should be balanced with appropriate educational provision and there should be clear evidence of consistency and continuity in the way that children are responded to by both teachers and child-care staff. Inspection of the educational arrangements is however subject to the Education Acts and outside the scope of the social services.

The co-ordination of child-care and teaching will require a planned approach. It is important that the educational and residential care arrangements complement each other and that physical provision is matched by recognition of individual children's emotional and personal relationships with each other and with staff.

4.6 Elderly people

4.6.1 General principles

The majority of places in residential homes are taken up by elderly people who have lived a full and active life in other settings. Unlike other client groups they are likely to have experienced a normal life prior to admission. Within one home, age may vary by as much as 30 years, though most people will be over 75. Personalities, interests, tastes, accustomed lifestyle and levels of physical and mental health will be extremely diverse. Indeed, often the only common characteristic of residents will be that they are not able to go on living independently or do not wish to do so.

Thus, residential homes catering for older people should put maximum emphasis on enabling residents to manage their own lives to the greatest attainable extent and so make it possible for them to maintain their dignity, their independence and their previous lifestyle. Allowances should be made for personal idiosyncracies which become exaggerated in old age.

The way elderly people are addressed and the use of names generally is important; staff should always use residents' names formally, attaching Mr., Mrs. or Miss unless invited to use a first name. 'Nicknames' should never be given to people by staff. Personal care needs to be offered discreetly and tactfully and not in a way which discourages self-help or the exercise of personal choice and autonomy. Routines should fit round the needs and wishes of residents as far as possible, and should not hinder the free use of private rooms; and staff should ensure that any nightly checks do not invade privacy unnecessarily and are undertaken in a sensitive manner. The layout, decor and furnishing of the home should be designed to minimise confusion and to facilitate mobility.

4.6.2 Elderly people with mental illness

The principles of good care are equally applicable to elderly residents who show signs of mental ill health. The first essential is to try to ensure that the causes of such symptoms are diagnosed and any necessary treatment given. Many kinds of physical illness can give rise to an acute confusional state, as can over-sedation or other inappropriate medication. Depressive illness is very common in old age and can easily be mistaken for dementia, and delusional symptoms can develop in an otherwise intact personality. All these conditions can be cured or alleviated and the proprietor has a responsibility to see that no such illness is ignored.

Some symptoms may persist however, and some illnesses which cause confusion, such as dementia of the Alzheimer type and dementia arising from a failure of blood supply to the brain, cannot be cured and may be progressive, but staff can help greatly by consistent and patient support. This should include regular toiletting and consistent encouragement to carry out familiar activities and self-care tasks. Talking to residents about the past and about present reality is also an important element in the caring process. Severe dementia does of course reduce capacity for autonomous decision-making, but considerable areas of choice and freedom can still be left open to the individual when these do not cause serious risk to the resident or nuisance to others. When direction or control is necessary, it should be by means of tactful and sympathetic supervision and distraction. Physical restraint may constitute an assault and should be avoided except in the most urgent circumstances and in the interests of immediate safety. Any restraint should be temporary and medical advice must be sought at once. Restraint by sedation can only be applied by a medical practitioner.

Such care is recognised to be a skilled and difficult task and staff will need support and training in understanding the needs of such residents and the effect of their presence which may be felt by others in the home. It is a duty of managers to see that such support and training is made available to the staff, and they should be able to call on a community psychiatric nurse and on a psycho-geriatrician and other members of his team for the assessment, advice and treatment services needed to help provide good and supportive care.

4.6.3 Special aids and care

Particular consideration needs to be given to the provision of communal facilities, personal aids and the sort of assistance which will minimise immobility, lack of capacity for self care and sensory loss. Illness should not be regarded as inevitable and untreatable in later life. It is important that any changing or developing condition should be brought to the attention of the resident's GP for diagnosis and treatment; incontinence, for example, may be cured or alleviated. Clear thought needs to be given to means of ensuring that people with acute or terminal illness receive not only the physical, but also the personal, attention appropriate to their needs and beliefs.

4.7 People recovering from drug addiction and alcohol abuse

4.7.1 Introduction

In addition to the general principles which apply to all residential care homes, other factors should also be taken into account when the aim of the home or hostel is to provide accommodation for the recuperation and rehabilitation of people with alcohol or drug or solvent abuse problems. The organisation of the home should be designed to achieve this aim and to return the individual to the community. This is a process which may require the imposition of a restrictive regime for which the informal consent of the resident should be obtained prior to admission. Failure to comply with the regime may result in expulsion.

4.7.2 General principles

Before admission an explanation of all the rules and regulations, especially those which modify residents' rights and freedoms, should be given, along with full details of any fees payable. There should be provision for receiving and dealing with complaints from residents, and residents' right to confidentiality should be ensured.

Appropriate arrangements should be made to ensure that all residents have opportunities for physical exercise, remedial education, where necessary, and a variety of leisure activities. In many cases residents will play a significant part in the maintenance and upkeep of the home. Whatever the regime they should, within clearly explained guidelines, be able to communicate by mail, have reasonable access to a telephone, and be able to receive visitors. The need to prevent the introduction of alcohol or illicit or injurious drugs into the residential care home should be balanced against the need to treat residents with respect.

Arrangements should be made to ensure that adequate space is available for recreational, communal and therapeutic activities. Where bedrooms are shared, whether as an element of a therapeutic regime or through necessity, opportunities for privacy should be safeguarded.

4.7.3 Staff and management

It is common and acceptable practice for people with a previous history of alcohol or drug addiction to be employed on the staff of residential care homes for people with similar problems. Such staff have usually completed a period of residence in a rehabilitation house. In these cases, it is desirable for staff either to have undertaken training or to have been employed elsewhere over a period of at least one year since completing rehabilitation or ceasing drug misuse. In-service training should be provided for all staff.

A clearly defined management structure should be established and understood by everyone concerned. Arrangements should be made to include representatives from the health, probation and social services, either as members of any management committee which is established, or as professional advisers to the home.

4.7.4 Health care

Residents should be registered with a local general medical practitioner; it may also be appropriate to retain the services of a consultant psychiatrist, or obtain other specialist clinical cover.

4.7.5 Residents subject to probation or supervision orders

Many people recovering from alcohol or drug abuse will be subject to a probation or supervision order. Arrangements for regular access to clients by the supervising probation officer should be agreed. Where appropriate, arrangements should be agreed for the appointment of a liaison probation officer. The liaison probation officer or supervising probation officer should be included in any decisions which might affect his or her clients' continued residence in the home.

5   Staff

5.1   Introduction

People who live in residential care homes are often vulnerable, both physically and emotionally. Staff will be required to carry out personal and potentially embarrassing intimate services for residents and will need special qualities to provide this service sensitively and tactfully. Such qualities will include personal warmth and patience and a responsiveness to and respect for the needs of the individual. Staff need to be able to provide competent and tactful care whilst supporting each person in maintaining and extending skills and self-care abilities. An understanding of the special emotional and/ or physical needs of the residents, and the skills necessary to provide for those needs in an efficient manner, is also required.

If residents are to receive a satisfactory standard of care, it is important that the staff see themselves as a consistent team with shared aims, each member providing his or her own input to fulfil complementary roles. A balance of staff will therefore need to be appointed to match the residents' needs, as outlined in the proprietor's statement for the home.

5.2   Staff selection

The selection of good staff is critical to the running of every home and must be undertaken carefully. Staff at all levels will need to demonstrate the right degree of knowledge, skills and experience relevant to their jobs, and in many of the senior and supervisory posts this will include the necessity for qualifications. It is also most important that staff should show appropriate attitudes to the clients, and those responsible for making appointments should interview candidates carefully and take up at least two relevant references. Wherever possible these should be from previous employers or people who have supervised relevant voluntary work undertaken by applicants, rather than character references from friends. In relation to all care staff, but senior staff in particular, it will be important to check that the applicant's curriculum vitae does not conceal unsatisfactory conduct. Prospective employees must disclose *all* previous convictions, and employers should give warning that these should include convictions 'otherwise spent'. The Rehabilitation of Offenders Act does not apply in the case of residential care staff; this is explained more fully in Annexe 1, p. 79.

5.3 Staffing establishments

There are four main groups of staff which need to be considered in developing the staff team:

Managerial and day care staff
Night care staff
Ancillary staff
Specialist staff.

Proprietors will be required to demonstrate that they have considered the residents' needs in relation to all four groups in drawing up their staffing proposals. The following paragraph is a brief guide — the subject is discussed in detail in *Staffing ratios in residential homes* published by the Residential Care Association. Upper levels of staffing in housing association shared accommodation, including hostels, are set out in the Housing Corporation's supplement on shared housing.

Staffing proposals should include the numbers of staff, their designations and duties, their gradings or salaries attached to posts, and the types of qualifications, experience and training which will be expected for each post. It is important to indicate the balance between part-time and full-time posts since part-time work allows for more flexible deployment while full-time posts tend to improve consistency and continuity of care. Job descriptions will be required for all posts, and all staff should be provided with the relevant written job description upon appointment. In larger homes there may be scope for some posts to be specialist (e.g. bursar), but in smaller homes staff may carry a wider variety of responsibilities, including managerial work, client care, cooking and so on. In all cases, however, the expectation of staff should be clear at the time of appointment, and any changes of duty or role should be made clear to the member of staff in writing.

5.4 Managerial and social care staff

5.4.1 Minimum cover

In drawing up their management and social care staffing establishments, proprietors should consider two main factors. The first is the provision of minimum cover. A unit where residents are fairly independent, for example, may be left unattended at times, but most homes must be staffed round the clock. In those where the work is more demanding, either physically or in terms of residents' behaviour, minimum staffing levels will be higher, and generally two staff will be needed at any one time where adults have to be lifted.

As a rule of thumb, with allowance made for time off, holidays and some illness, a home needs to employ 3.5 staff to provide one person on day duty. Where at least two staff are needed on duty at all times, the minimum cover would therefore demand $3.5 \times 2 = 7.00$ staff. These figures are given in full-time equivalents, but could be filled by part-time staff, or a mixture of full- and part-timers.

These approximate minimum staffing figures are based upon a full-time working week of 36 to 40 hours. Where proprietors, managers or other senior staff are resident and are prepared to be available on call for longer periods, minimum staffing calculations may take this into account, but proprietors must always be able to show that there will be adequate cover when resident staff are absent, and that resident staff do not have excessive demands placed upon them. Proprietors' dependent relatives also living on the premises should be taken into account when cover is assessed. Where married couples are the proprietors or are employed, care should be taken to ensure that these couples have reasonable time off together each week and for holidays, and that they are not under pressure to forego this right for lack of staffing.

While the minimum cover is designed to cope with the type of problems which may arise at any time in the home, there are also peaks and troughs in the residents' demand for staff support and help. Peaks include getting up, meal times, activities and going to bed; troughs include times when residents are out of the building and rest periods. It is important, therefore, not only to provide minimum cover but also to deploy staff to offer additional support at peak periods. The employment of part-time staff can enable such deployment to be flexible without causing problems such as split shifts for full-timers.

5.4.2 Total staff required

The second main factor in the calculation of day care staffing is the degree of need presented by the client group and the consequent amount of staff time required. It is possible to estimate the number of care hours required per resident per annum and when these are totalled for a home, the number of staff needed can be worked out, once allowance is made for holidays, illness and other absences. Annexe 5 gives one possible approach to estimating the number of care hours required by residents. This approach gives the total staffing required for all managerial and care staff on day duties, inclusive of the minimum cover outlined above. Where an establishment is geared towards encouraging self care and participation in household tasks, no staffing reduction can be permitted as the staff help needed in the process is considerable, but clearly residents who become increasingly independent will need less support.

In calculating the care time that staff can provide to clients, allowance has to be made for leave, sickness, training, staff meetings and other activities. Where senior staff are involved in client selection, recruitment of staff, fund-raising and additional extraneous duties, further allowance will need to be made. In general, a full-time employee can provide about 1500 hours of care time per annum.

5.5   Night staffing

Night staffing requirements will depend upon the mobility and lucidity of residents on the one hand, and the type of handling problems anticipated on the other. Where residents require lifting, for example, two members of staff are required, regardless of the size of the home. In order to calculate the staffing required, an establishment of 2.5 full-time equivalents is sufficient to provide one person on duty minimum cover. Where wakeful staff on duty are not sufficiently experienced and trained, it will be necessary for senior staff to sleep on call on the premises.

5.6   Ancillary staff

Ancillary staffing includes staff not primarily engaged to undertake managerial or social care roles, but this should not under-estimate the value of their contact with residents or their therapeutic role. In large establishments the management of ancillary staff is likely to require experience and a different set of skills. While no specific guidelines are offered for the numbers of such staff, proprietors should consider the following tasks.

5.6.1 Cooking

In some establishments residents are expected to participate in the cooking, while in others it is undertaken by care staff to help create a homely atmosphere, or, in larger establishments, by full-time cooks. The approach should be determined by the overall aim of the home, and appropriate training made available to ensure that residents obtain a varied, balanced diet that also reflects their individual wishes.

5.6.2 Laundry work and needlework

In large homes or where incontinence presents major problems, consideration may be given to the appointment of staff to deal solely with laundry. Needlework may be undertaken by residents or care staff, but there may be homes where a needleworker should be appointed to care for residents' clothes. It is important in both laundering and needlework that residents' clothing should be well treated, since carelessness may not only damage the clothes but seriously upset residents and their families who see it as a sign of institutional treatment. Some clothes may also need adjustment for handicapped people.

5.6.3 Domestic work

Communal areas will normally be cleaned by paid staff, even in homes where residents are encouraged to clean their private rooms. Old buildings are sometimes more difficult to clean and will require extra time.

5.6.4	**Gardening and maintenance**	This work may be carried out by proprietors, care staff, residents or outside contractors. In some circumstances, however, staff may be appointed to carry out this work, since good maintenance is important for the comfort of residents, especially when they are dependent on the maintenance of heating systems, hot water supplies, other household systems and the efficient functioning of aids with which the home is equipped.
5.6.5	**Clerical work and administration**	It is important that both the social care and managerial aspects of the home are properly backed by clerical and administrative staff, to ensure that clients' records, correspondence, appointments, and financial records and general administration, are kept up to date, without using senior managerial time inappropriately.

5.7 Specialists

The fourth group of staff to be considered are the specialists who may be required to provide advice or services beyond the skills of the home staff. Many of these may be available through the National Health Service, such as community nurses, community psychiatric nurses, physiotherapists, chiropodists, doctors, dentists, and consultants, including psychiatrists. Others, such as social workers and occupational therapists, may be available as part of the local authority social services support. However, some may need to be considered as part of the paid staffing, such as specialist advisers acting in a consultant capacity to the home. Proprietors should demonstrate that they have considered the range of specialist services the residents may require, or that the staff may need in order to fulfil their roles, and they will have to show how these services are to be provided and whether or not they are to be paid for by the proprietor.

5.8 Management, supervision and support

Having drawn up the staffing establishment required, proprietors should ensure that managerial structures, communications systems and staff supervision are sufficient to enable the staff to undertake their duties. It is not acceptable for a home to be left in the control of a person with insufficient training and experience. The staffing establishment and rota system therefore need to be arranged so that there are enough senior staff and that they are suitably deployed to give the cover required to meet the home's stated aims. Homes should also enable staff to develop their own careers. Staff induction training, manuals of guidance, in-house training, staff meetings and individual supervision all require to be considered carefully and laid out in detail. The extent to which staff need these forms of support will depend upon the complexity and stress involved in the work, but in the event of crises and enquiries, proprietors may well have to demonstrate that the support they offered staff was sufficient. Good working relationships will be enhanced by the involvement of all levels of staff in discussions about the running of the home; this should include encouragement to residents to offer their views.

5.9   Training, qualifications and experience

The responsible person in charge of the day-to-day running of the residential care home should normally have not less than one year's experience at a senior level in a residential care home and/or a qualification recognised by the registration authority as appropriate for the stated aim of the establishment. He must be able to demonstrate an ability to undertake those tasks required to administer and manage the establishment successfully. Residential care homes should enable and encourage staff to undertake training and the registration authority should provide assistance under the terms of registration for training. It is sometimes easier to provide training in the setting in which the staff are employed and many registration authorities are initiating such schemes. Such training should be seen as an integral part of the running of the establishment, and emphasis should be given to timing, arrangement of staffing rotas to allow training, and relief staff cover. Staff should be referred to qualifying and non-qualifying courses, validated by the Central Council for Education and Training in Social Work, and to other relevant agencies and personnel dealing with training of residential care staff. The registration authorities should ensure that all homes are made aware of such training opportunities. The importance and associated costs of training of all staff employed in residential care homes will need to be fully reflected when assessing the level of charges to residents.

5.10   Volunteers

If people undertake voluntary work in residential homes, the responsible person in charge should ensure that they are aware of the stated aims and philosophy of the home, and that a description of the role of each volunteer is provided. Staff should be made aware of the particular contribution expected from all volunteers.

The role of the registration authority in the management and inspection of private and voluntary residential care homes

Responsibilities of the local authority

Legislation has laid responsibility on the local authority to be the agency responsible for the standards of residential care. The registration authority is required to ensure that the purposes and aims of residential establishments are clearly set out and the standards of care they offer match these aims and objectives. In addition registration authorities have a duty to ensure that the best possible quality of life for residents is achieved. Members of staff appointed by registration authorities to undertake inspection of residential care homes, give advice to staff and be responsible to the registration authority for recommendations concerning registration, should be knowledgeable and skilled in communicating with proprietors from a wide range of backgrounds. They should have sufficient experience and status to receive the respect of colleagues and staff of homes alike. The demands made upon the officers engaged in this work are such that the registration authority should ensure that other, unrelated demands made on them are kept to a minimum. In at least one region of the country registration officers have set up an association which holds regular seminars and meetings. These are generally agreed to be beneficial. Other regions may well consider doing this.

Pre-registration

The response to initial enquiries from prospective proprietors ought to set out the registration requirements in general terms. This is best done in the form of a guide, listing key documents relating to the registration process. A copy of this Code of Practice should be included together with a list of or extracts from the following:—

1 Relevant extracts from the *Registered Homes Act 1984* and the regulations under that Act relating to the registration of residential care homes.

2 Memorandum of guidance on arrangements for health care as specified in DHSS Circular HC(77)25,LAC(77)13, Welsh Office Circular 117/77, WHC(77)30 dated July 1977, together with any code of practice on general health matters agreed and published locally.

3 *Food Hygiene (General) Regulations, 1970.*

4 *Fire Precautions as Agreed in Existing Residential Homes.* DHSS Circular LAC(77)6, Welsh Office Circular 62/77 together with Annexe A and Annexe B dated 6th April 1977.

Home Office, *Draft Guide to Fire Precautions in Existing Resi-dential Care Premises.* DHSS Circular LAC(83)4, Januar 1983.

5   A statement emphasising the requirements for consultatio with the registration authority before any building alter ations or adaptations are carried out, or in the event of ; change of ownership subsequent to registration.

6   Copies of Hazard Notices issued by the DHSS and the Welsh Office.

7   Notes of guidance on specific matters which may have beer formulated locally. These might include, for example, note: highlighting the danger regarding the use of portable calo gas heating appliances or a policy statement about the methods of controlling disruptive residents in children': homes or homes for mentally handicapped people.

8   A statement of the registration authority's policy in relatior to the services and facilities to be provided locally and the extent to which standards required are based upon *Buildinç Notes* and other relevant publications.

9   An indication of the staffing requirements and criteria whicl are applied by the registration authority.

10   Information regarding County and District Council anc DHSS local offices, including the location of Area Socia Services offices.

11   Bibliography to include current publications on census anc research data relevant to residential care.

12   Specimen forms relating to:
Drugs administration
Residents' records forms
Financial record sheets (residents' financial affairs)
Suggested guidelines for a model prospectus/brochure.

13   A map showing the location of existing private and volun-tary homes situated within the area of the registration auth-ority, together with information about any local associatior offering support to managers and/ or residents.

14   Application for registration form (see Annexe 3, Model 1).

15   A statement explaining situations in which dual registratior with the health authority is likely to be required.

When issuing the registration guide or file, it is desirable that the registration authority includes an offer of an interview/ discussion with the intending proprietor. At the interview stage the aims and objectives of the proposed residential care home can be fully discussed, in the context of the over-all situation within the local area. The representative of the registration authority will be able to advise the various steps to be taken (e.g. the need to approach the fire authority) as well as outlining the policies of the registration authority.

In areas where the registration authority receives a parti-cularly large number of enquiries about registration and opening a residential home, seminars organised by registration staff can be an effective medium for the exchange of information. Registration staff should ensure that representatives from the planning authority/ building control, environmental health and fire prevention departments are involved at all stages of the pre-registration/ registration processes. It may, on occasions, be necessary for registration staff and representatives from other agencies to make joint visits to sites where the suitability of premises to be used as residential care homes is being assessed.

6.3 Finance and the placement of residents in private and voluntary homes

As part of the pre-registration consultation, the financial implications of establishing a new residential care home should be explained. The authority's own policy regarding sponsorship should be conveyed to all new applicants. Local authority committees are responsible for setting and approving their own budgets, allocating finance to cover the costs of placing clients in private and voluntary homes. Where authorities do provide sponsorship, a client can be placed in residential care either within or outside the authority's administrative area. Normally the address where the client is 'ordinarily resident' decides which authority is responsible for sponsorship. The role of the local offices of the DHSS and the application of supplementary benefit should be explained. Similarly, the responsibility of residents in connection with their own financial affairs should be emphasised.

Voluntary homes or hostels which are registered Housing Associations may attract funding from the Housing Corporation in the form of grants, management allowances or other benefits. Specialist advice is available from the National Federation of Housing Associations.

6.4 The suitability of applicants for registration

Registration authorities should ensure that all prospective proprietors/ managers of homes possess some relevant qualifications or have some proven experience of employment within residential care. A prospective proprietor should also be able to demonstrate competence in and understanding of financial projections and budgeting. He should show that he possesses a business-like approach which will ensure that any new private home will be managed on a secure financial basis which will not put the future welfare of residents at risk. Where the registration authority receives applications for registration from voluntary organisations the local, regional or national chairman, secretary or like person of the management committee of the home is registered, together with the home's manager or administrator. The registration authority should ascertain the actual and legal divisions of responsibility within the organisation. Notification of any changes of those personnel should be made to the authority once the home is registered.

The registration authority should ensure that a check is made on the DHSS national list of people who have been de-registered. When many applications are received from people who have no specific experience of residential care or of managing a small business, the registration authority might consider setting up, in conjunction with a local college of education, a part-time introduction course which prepares them for the task. DHSS offers a consultancy service to local authorities in relation to staff who work with children in residential care homes. In the case of voluntary and charitable bodies, the applicants for registration are likely to be the honorary officers of the association, or the honorary officers of a management committee with delegated powers. It should be recognised that the backgrounds and skills of such voluntary management bodies will vary greatly, and where previous experience of managing a home is lacking, advice on training, costings and staff appointments may be necessary, and welcomed.

6.5 The registration process

Throughout the registration process, registration staff will need to be available to monitor progress and preparations for the opening of the home. Advice may need to be given to proprietors about the initial selection of residents, selection of staff, preparation of a home brochure, and to ensure that the registration requirements agreed initially are being implemented. Where the home is likely to receive residents placed by the local or other social services department, the role and contribution of the social worker needs to be fully explained. Care should be given to explaining the needs of special client groups and those who may be subject to additional legal requirements. Prior to the opening of a new home, registration staff should inform proprietors or home managers about the full range of services available in their particular area, and to which their residents are entitled from the social services department, the health authority and the education authority. The provision of aids for disabled people, specialist advice for blind and deaf people and information on community health services, are some of the services that need to be noted.

6.6 Opportunities for further training for proprietors, managers and care staff

The registration authority may wish to offer proprietors, managers and senior staff from private and voluntary homes places on courses and training programmes organised for staff employed in residential care within the public sector. The value of training which is jointly organised with the health authority should be considered, especially when the homes are required to be dually registered. Information about alternative sources of training should also be made available.

5.7 Registration approval

Prospective proprietors/ managers should be reminded that there are penalties for operating an un-registered home and no residents should be admitted until a certificate of registration is issued. Certificates of registration should be issued as soon as practicable.

5.8 Change of proprietor or manager of a residential care home

Once the initial certificate of registration has been issued, proprietors should notify the registration authority of any intended change of ownership. Registrations are not automatically transferred to new proprietors or managers. New applications must be lodged and references taken up. Residents and, where they wish it, their relatives should be fully informed of any changes. This is particularly crucial where there has been a close relationship formed between the proprietor/ manager and the residents in his care.

5.9 Change of facilities or objectives

If any change should occur or is planned in the facilities or objectives described in the brochure, the registration authority must be informed so that the validity of registration can be considered in the new circumstances. The brochure should be altered so that it describes the new situation accurately.

6.10 Dual registration (see also 2.7.6)

When a proprietor wishes or is required to apply for dual registration as a residential care home and nursing home, the applicant must be able to satisfy the registration authority that the requirements of the Regulations will be met within the home, and should satisfy both authorities that the recommendations of this Code will be followed.

6.11 Inspection

Following initial registration, a visit of inspection should be made within the first three months of the home becoming established, or when a new manager of a home has been appointed.

Thereafter, there is a statutory responsibility placed on the registration authority to carry out at least one annual inspection visit. Registration authorities are free to continue a policy of regular visiting at more frequent intervals. In the case of dual registration, the health authority has a duty to carry out inspections twice a year. In this situation it may be advisable for the registration authority to do likewise. Joint visits could foster valuable cooperation and avoid misunderstanding. There will be occasions, however, when more frequent, unannounced visits will be essential. For example, a visit would be necessary following an anonymous or specific complaint made to the authority about poor standards of care in a home, or, where a proprietor or company owns several homes, the registration authority may need to satisfy itself that the homes' managers are receiving adequate supervision and support. Inspections should focus on the quality of life and care of the residents and give special attention to standards of management. Normally it should be possible for inspections to be conducted in a way which is seen to be constructive by managers and staff of the home. Recognition should be given to innovative and good residential care practice. For a formal review inspection, the check list (see Annexe 3 Model 2) should be used as a guide to aid this process, but should not be seen as a substitute for discussion with the proprietor or manager in reviewing the objectives of the home and how the care of the residents can be enhanced.

At the formal annual review any change of circumstances affecting the registration will need to be identified. The authority should ensure that a report on the formal review is sent to the proprietor and the manager, drawing attention to any specific points of consultation and specifying any variation in the registration requirements. Care should be taken to ensure that courtesy, diplomacy and tact are used in inspecting individual residents' private rooms. The proprietor or manager of the home must make it possible for the inspection officer to spend some time in private with individual residents.

6.12 Complaints procedures

The majority of complaints regarding the management of a home will normally be satisfactorily resolved by the proprietor or home manager and there will be no need for the registration authority to be involved. Each home should have its own established complaints procedure and this should be outlined in the home's brochure/prospectus.

When complaints cannot be resolved internally, the registration authority should be informed of the complaint. All complaints regarding a specific home should initially be made in writing to the registration authority, giving details of any action already taken and with whom the matter has been discussed. The registration authority will then take the necessary steps to investigate the complaint and arrange to interview the proprietor/manager, resident and all other people relevant to the specific complaint. Following the investigation/ interview, a letter should be sent to the proprietor and manager, resident and the complainant stating the outcome and specifying any action.

6.13 De-registration

In circumstances where a registration authority is considering de-registration of a home, registration staff should ensure that the proprietor and manager are notified of the intention to de-register, prior to the implementation of the statutory procedures. At an appropriate stage, residents, next of kin, or key supporters should be notified that the registration authority is being recommended to take such action. It is also essential to notify any sponsoring agencies that it may be necessary for them to make alternative accommodation arrangements for residents.

The Registered Homes Act 1984 provides for appeals against decisions of registration authorities to be made to Registered Homes Tribunals. Such appeals must be made within 28 days of the decision being notified. Registration authorities should make proprietors aware of their right to appeal and the procedure to be followed.

6.14 Consumer advice

The registration authority must make available for inspection a list of all private and voluntary homes currently registered in its area. Many authorities have also found it helpful to publish a more detailed list of registered homes describing individual characteristics of homes and specific services provided, i.e. levels of staffing and medical cover provided within the home. General information can also be given on how to obtain advice about financial assistance towards the cost of accommodation, and on the difference between a private and voluntary home and between a residential care home and a nursing home. Enquirers and prospective residents should also be reminded to request a copy of the home's brochure when seeking initial information from a proprietor or manager.

7 Summary of recommendations— a check list

In order to clarify the status of items in this check list, the word 'must' has been reserved for legal requirements. The legal basis of these requirements lies outside the Code.

Para no.
(page no.)

Social care
Admission procedures

1   All homes should produce a brochure setting out the aims of the establishment and the facilities which it intends to provide.   2.1.1 (18

2   Intending residents should be able to visit a home prior to admission and to be visited by someone from the home in the place where they are living.   2.1.2 (18

3   The admission of residents on a short-term basis into a home should not disrupt or diminish the quality of life of longer-term residents.   2.1.3 (18

4   The first two months after a resident enters a home on a long-term basis should be agreed by both parties as a recognised trial period.   2.1.4 (18

5   At the end of the trial period, the ability of the home to meet the needs of the resident should be fully considered by the resident, the proprietor and any key supporters.   2.1.5 (19

6   Subsequent regular reviews should take place, in order to plan future health and social care for the resident.   2.1.6 (19

7   The resident and a key supporter should normally be present during the reviews.   2.1.6 (19

8   Residents should be encouraged to bring personal possessions, including furniture, into a home.   2.1.7 (19

9   Residents' personal possessions should be treated with respect, and any valuable items noted. Unobtrusive procedures for the recording of major additions and deletions should be established.   2.1.7 (19

10   Residents should be helped to buy their own clothing and should never be supplied with clothing from a communal pool.   2.1.8 (19

Terms and conditions of residence

11   All residents, and where necessary their sponsor as well, should be given in writing a clear statement of the terms under which the accommodation is offered.   2.2.1 (19)

12   Homes should be made aware of health factors affecting the type of care required. These should include the prospective resident's current medical condition and prognosis, together with any relevant social circumstances.   2.2.2 (20)

13	Information of this nature should be provided with the consent of the resident, and treated in the strictest confidence.	2.2.2 (20)

General administration

14	Records which the home is required to keep must be kept in a secure place and treated as confidential. Such records must be available for inspection by the registration authority.	2.3.1 (20)
15	Domestic routines in the home should aim to meet the needs and preferences of the resident rather than administrative convenience.	2.3.2 (21)
16	Rules relating to residents should be kept to a minimum.	2.3.3 (21)
17	Residents should be encouraged to maintain their independence within the home, recognising that this may involve a degree of responsible risk-taking.	2.3.3 (21)
18	Residents should be involved as much as possible in making decisions concerning the way in which the home is run.	2.3.4 (21)
19	Residents should be addressed in the manner they have chosen.	2.3.5 (21)
20	Professional advice and guidance from the registration authority should be sought when a resident's ability to make decisions or exercise choice appears to be in doubt.	2.3.6 (21)
21	All complaints should be treated seriously and recorded.	2.3.7 (22)
22	Residents should be made aware that they have the right to refer any unresolved complaint to the registration authority.	2.3.7 (22)
23	Any infringement of this Code of Practice should constitute grounds for a complaint.	2.3.7 (22)
24	Residents should normally have access to their personal records maintained by the home.	2.3.8 (22)
25	When information is provided about, or derived from, a third party it should not be disclosed to a resident without the consent of that third party.	2.3.8 (22)
26	Information about a child should not be given to parents or guardians without the child's consent, unless the child is precluded by age or mental impairment from giving informed consent.	2.3.8 (22)
27	Information may be withheld from the resident only in exceptional circumstances and after most careful assessment. Such a decision should be made at senior level within the home, and the resident may appeal to the registration authority.	2.3.8 (22)

Security of tenure

28	If there is any doubt about security of tenure, residents should be referred to a local Citizens Advice Bureau or the local Law Society.	2.4 (23)

Privacy and personal autonomy

29   It is recommended that residents in long-term care should have their own room, unless they prefer otherwise.   2.5.1 (23)

30   The right to privacy in residents' own rooms should be respected.   2.5.1 (23)

31   Where rooms are shared, personal space for each resident should be provided and privacy ensured by the use of room dividers and other furniture.   2.5.1 (23)

32   Bedroom and sitting room temperatures should be maintained at similar levels.   2.5.1 (23)

33   Residents should be able to meet whom they wish in private, either in their own room, or in other comfortable accommodation.   2.5.1 (23)

34   Residents should be encouraged to pursue existing interests and acquire new ones.   2.5.2 (23)

35   Residents' mobility should be maintained by encouraging walks, outside visits and social activity.   2.5.2 (23)

36   All residents should be enabled to make use of community facilities.   2.5.2 (23)

37   Involvement in political and religious activities should be respected, provided it does not interfere unduly with others.   2.5.2 (23)

38   Visitors should be welcome at all reasonable times.   2.5.3 (24)

39   A resident's right to refuse to see a visitor should be respected.   2.5.3 (24)

40   If a proprietor decides to exclude a resident's visitor, he should record the fact, and be able to justify this action to the registration authority.   2.5.3 (24)

41   The involvement of suitable volunteers to befriend isolated residents is to be encouraged.   2.5.4 (24)

Financial affairs

42   Adults who are likely to be permanent residents should be encouraged to make a will prior to admission to the home.   2.6.1 (25)

43   Proprietors or staff should not normally act as witnesses to any resident's will. In no circumstances should the proprietor or any member of staff become an executor of any resident's will.   2.6.1 (25)

44   If a resident's incompetence to make a will is confirmed by a medical practitioner, consideration should be given to contacting the Court of Protection.   2.6.1 (25)

45   It should be the publicly-known practice of a home to decline all personal gifts from residents, except for small token presents. If a resident insists, independent advice, if possible from the registration authority, should be sought.   2.6.2 (25)

46   The acceptance of gratuities by staff should not be permitted.   2.6.3 (26)

47	Residents should be made aware of their responsibility for the safe-keeping of money and valuables, and of any insurance provided by the home which covers this. They should be advised to take out any further insurance which may be needed.	2.6.3 (26)
48	The home must have a secure facility, with limited access by a responsible person, for the storage of residents' valuables. Receipts should be given to depositors.	2.6.3 (26)
49	The home should also keep a permanent register of deposits and withdrawals.	2.6.3 (26)
50	In the case of temporary or permanent incapacity of a resident to safeguard his possessions, the agent acting on his behalf should undertake the responsibility (see 51–54).	2.6.3 (26)
51	A resident may appoint a relative, friend or someone over 18 in the community to act as his agent in the handling of his finances.	2.6.4 (26)
52	In the absence of someone known to the resident, the registration authority should be asked to recommend someone to act as agent. References for agents should be sought, and all names of individuals and organisations acting as agents should be lodged with the registration authority. Only in exceptional circumstances should the proprietor or manager assume the role of agent.	2.6.4 (26)
53	A resident wishing to delegate more extensive powers to act on his behalf may execute a power of attorney. No-one connected with the home should be appointed an attorney.	2.6.4 (26)
54	When a qualified medical practitioner has assessed a resident as mentally unable to manage his financial affairs, and the value of assets warrants it, careful consideration should be given to placing the resident under the jurisdiction of the Court of Protection.	2.6.5 (27)
55	In the case of children, guidance and education in the handling of personal money is good practice.	2.6.6 (28)
56	Proprietors and staff should not become involved in the handling and management of residents' monies. They should be able to draw the attention of the registration authority to any concern they may have about particular problems of a resident's finances.	2.6.7 (28)

Health care

57	All residents have the right of access to health and remedial services provided in the community.	2.7.1 (28)
58	Homes have the right of access to community health resources for their residents.	2.7.1 (28)
59	No medical treatment must be given to a resident without his valid consent except where the law permits in cases of	2.7.2 (28)

life-threatening emergencies, or under the terms of the Mental Health Act 1983.

60 When a resident's ability to give valid consent is restricted by inability to understand the language, every effort must be made to explain the nature of the treatment and to gain consent through the use of an interpreter.   2.7.2 (28)

61 Children under 16 may be able to consent to or refuse treatment. Where they cannot do so by reason of age or mental impairment, parents or those *in loco parentis* may do so, subject to the Court's powers to take action in the child's best interests.   2.7.2 (28)

62 Only household remedies should be given without a doctor's prescription.   2.7.3 (29)

63 Residents who are deemed able to retain and administer their own medication should be encouraged to do so, and have a secure place to keep it in.   2.7.3 (29)

64 Drugs for which the proprietor is responsible must be kept in a secure place, be individually labelled, and administered only by the trained responsible person authorised by the proprietor. A record must be kept of drugs received and administered by the home.   2.7.3 (29)

65 A resident's failure to take prescribed drugs which are held by the proprietor should be reported to the resident's medical practitioner.   2.7.3 (29)

66 The proprietor should take responsibility for ensuring that staff are trained in the administration of drugs.   2.7.3 (29)

67 Medication must never be administered as a means of social control.   2.7.3 (29)

Dying and death

68 When a home has admitted a resident with an assurance of 'care till death', the use of external sources of care, such as the community nursing, or hospice nursing service, is strongly recommended.   2.7.5 (30)

69 Intensive or terminal care should be given in a resident's own room and not in any special unit.   2.7.5 (30)

70 If a resident is aware he is dying, he should be consulted about his wishes on terminal care and funeral or cremation arrangements.   2.7.5 (30)

71 Contact should be made, if the resident wishes it, with the appropriate minister of religion.   2.7.5 (30)

72 When a resident is dying, the need for support to relatives, staff, and other residents should be recognised and met.   2.7.5 (30)

73 Local, cultural and religious customs surrounding the death of a resident should be observed.   2.7.5 (30)

74   Proprietors should ascertain at an early stage who will take   2.7.5 (30)
responsibility for a resident's property pending the proving of
a will.

Physical features

75   When considering whether there is reasonable and appropri-   3.1   (32)
ate accommodation and space, the registration authority will
refer to the appropriate Building Notes. In the case of
adapted premises, these should be flexibly interpreted.

76   Registering authorities should ensure that the location and   3.2   (32)
surrounding environment are suited to the aims of a home,
in the case of new applications.

77   The availability of local amenities, accessibility, health   3.2   (32)
services and public transport should be considerations in
granting registration.

78   The physical size of the building and the total number of   3.3   (32)
residents in each social grouping within it shall be important
considerations in deciding whether to grant registration.

79   The stated aims of the establishment should determine what   3.4   (32)
is meant by reasonable accommodation and space and such
accommodation should conform to the relevant Building
Notes for particular client groups.

80   Communal rooms in a home should be arranged to allow   3.4   (32)
residents to follow their chosen hobbies or interests. Where
there are children there should be room for homework to be
done.

81   The home should be decorated and furnished in a non-insti-   3.4   (32)
tutional manner.

82   Storage space for residents' luggage should be provided.   3.5   (33)

83   All residents' rooms should have at least one armchair, chest   3.5   (33)
of drawers, wardrobe facilities and table. There should be one
lockable piece of furniture.

84   In rooms for adults and older children, there should be   3.5   (33)
accessible power and light sockets. For younger children
these must not be easily accessible.

85   Residents should be allowed a choice of bedding, and it   3.5   (33)
should be ensured that such bedding is flame- and smoulder-
proof.

86   Floors in residents' rooms should be covered in non-slip   3.5   (33)
materials.

87   Residents should be able to have their names outside their   3.5   (33)
doors, if wished, and where possible letter boxes and locks
should be provided on the doors.

88   There should be a private washbasin within each bedroom.   3.6   (34)

89	Washing areas in bedrooms should be screened to provide privacy.	3.6	(34
90	There should be an overall ratio of one toilet to four residents.	3.6	(34
91	One bathroom to eight residents should be the minimum provided.	3.6	(34
92	The ratios of toilets and bathrooms to residents should not include those exclusively for staff use.	3.6	(34
93	The location and fittings of bathrooms and toilets should be planned to minimise the effects of disability of residents.	3.6	(34)
94	Equipment should be provided for residents who so wish to launder their personal clothing.	3.7	(34)

Diet and food preparation

95	Meals must be varied, properly served and nutritious, and should provide choice.	3.8	(34)
96	Ready-plated meals should be avoided.	3.8	(34)
97	The timing of meals should be flexible and provision made for residents to prepare snacks and drinks for themselves.	3.8	(34)
98	Attention to residents with eating difficulties should be given discreetly.	3.8	(34)
99	Homes should be prepared to cater for special diets, whether these are medically advised, of cultural, religious or philosophical significance or the result of strong preference.	3.8	(34)
100	Residents should never be deceived into eating foods they would not otherwise take.	3.8	(34)
101	Staff training should include the cultural and social importance of meals, their content and preparation.	3.8	(34)
102	Proprietors should ascertain residents' dietary needs on admission, seeking advice from the community dietician or religious advisers where necessary in order to meet these needs.	3.8	(34)

Client groups

| 103 | Irrespective of the client group, homes should understand the importance of recognising and responding to the needs of the individual residents and enabling them to achieve their maximum potential. | 4.1 | (36) |

Disabled people

| 104 | Disabled people should have normal opportunities to make informed choices and take risks. | 4.2.1 | (36) |
| 105 | The intimate personal needs of handicapped people should be met sensitively, always enabling them to retain autonomy and dignity. | 4.2.1 | (36) |

106	Staff should be trained to understand the communication needs and difficulties of residents suffering from sensory handicaps and speech disorders.	4.2.2 (37)
107	Accommodation should be adapted and aids provided to reduce the effects of disability.	4.2.3 (37)
108	The disabled person should be consulted about his needs and management of his disability.	4.2.4 (37)

Mentally ill people

109	Signs of institutionalisation in former long-stay hospital patients should be recognised and their special needs identified in making appropriate placements.	4.3.1 (37)
110	Staff should have the support and advice of relevant professions in the community.	4.3.2 (38)
111	Where a therapeutic regime limits autonomy, the resident should first be given a full explanation and agree to accept such limitations.	4.3.4 (38)
112	Provision of positive day-time activity is essential and may be met either in the home or community. The resources of specialist voluntary agencies should be considered.	4.3.5 (39)
113	In the case of a placement from hospital the registration authority should ensure that arrangements are agreed to cover after-care of the resident.	4.3.6 (39)

Mentally handicapped people

114	The home should create an enabling environment for mentally handicapped people, encouraging choice.	4.4.1 (40)
115	A full assessment of educational and social potential, and physical and emotional needs, should be available on admission.	4.4.2 (40)
116	Mentally handicapped residents should have access to a social worker or other suitable person to provide personal support.	4.4.3 (40)
117	Appropriate day-time occupation and education in the case of a child must be arranged and activities for adults should be provided.	4.4.4 (41)
118	Opportunities for suitable employment should be considered at regular reviews.	4.4.4 (41)

Children and young people

119	Proprietors and staff should be aware of reactions and behaviour patterns of child residents.	4.5.2 (42)
120	Staff should have an understanding of the significance of personal relationships between a child and care staff.	4.5.2 (42)
121	Children should be helped to understand the reality of their situation and their need to be in the home.	4.5.2 (42)

122	The recording of past events in a 'life story book' will be of major importance to most children.	4.5.3 (43)
123	Long-term goal planning should involve the child. Plans should not make unrealistic demands upon the child.	4.5.3 (43)
124	Controls and sanctions should not undermine the self-respect of children.	4.5.4 (43)
125	Intervention should be positive rather than negative, based on reward rather than punishment.	4.5.4 (43)
126	Restriction of contact with parents, food deprivation and other unacceptable sanctions should not be used.	4.5.4 (43)
127	All sanctions used to control bad behaviour must be recorded and this record must be available for inspection by authorised persons.	4.5.4 (43)
128	Parents should share and be responsible for decisions affecting the child whenever possible.	4.5.5 (44)
129	Care staff should be able to offer understanding and reassurance to parents.	4.5.5 (44)
130	Handicapped children have the same needs as other children and should have the same opportunities to develop their full potential.	4.5.6 (44)
131	Proprietors and staff should be made aware of specialist help available for handicapped children.	4.5.6 (44)
132	The child's legal status should be clearly identified on admission. Explanations should be given to the resident and staff of the effect of the legal status of a child resident and of restrictions imposed by orders of the court.	4.5.7 (44)
133	Proprietors must make suitable arrangements for the education of all children present.	4.5.8 (44)

Elderly people

134	The right of elderly residents to autonomy and choice should always be recognised.	4.6.1 (45)
135	The layout, decor and furnishing of the home should be designed to minimise confusion.	4.6.1 (45)
136	Staff should be trained to understand the needs of mentally and physically frail old people.	4.6.2 (46)
137	Community support and treatment services should be consulted in the care of mentally ill elderly people.	4.6.2 (46)
138	Physical restraint and control by sedation should not be used.	4.6.2 (46)

Drug addiction, alcohol and solvent abuse

139	Before admission the potential resident should have a full explanation of the regime and any rules which modify his freedom.	4.7.2 (47)

140	Admission should be subject to a contractual agreement.	4.7.2 (47)
141	Residents should be encouraged to participate in the day-to-day running of the home or hostel.	4.7.2 (47)
142	Within the limits of the regime, opportunities and space for privacy should be safeguarded.	4.7.2 (47)
143	In-service training should be provided for all staff.	4.7.3 (48)
144	Staff with a personal history of addiction should have undertaken training or have been employed elsewhere for at least one year after completing rehabilitation.	4.7.3 (48)
145	A clearly defined management structure should be agreed. Health, social services and probation service representatives should act as advisers or members of the management committee.	4.7.3 (48)
146	Where appropriate, the proprietor should retain the service of a consultant psychiatrist.	4.7.4 (48)
147	Where residents are subject to a supervision or probation order, arrangements for regular access to clients by probation officers must be agreed.	4.7.5 (48)

Staff

148	Staff qualities should include responsiveness to and respect for the needs of the individual.	5.1 (49)
149	Staff skills should match the residents' needs as identified in the objectives of the home.	5.1 (49)
150	Staff should have the ability to give competent and tactful care, whilst enabling residents to retain dignity and self-determination.	5.1 (49)
151	In the selection of staff at least two references should be taken up, where possible from previous employers.	5.2 (49)
152	Applicants' curriculum vitae should be checked and for this purpose employers should give warning that convictions otherwise spent should be disclosed.	5.2 (49)
153	Proprietors should consider residents' needs in relation to all categories of staff when drawing up staffing proposals.	5.3 (50)
154	Job descriptions will be required for all posts and staff should be provided with relevant job descriptions on appointment.	5.3 (50)
155	In small homes where staff carry a range of responsibilities, these must be clearly understood by staff.	5.3 (50)
156	Any change of role or duty should be made clear to the member of staff in writing.	5.3 (50)
157	Minimum staff cover should be designed to cope with residents' anticipated problems at any time.	5.4.1 (50)
158	Staff deployment should take account of periods of high demand.	5.4.1 (50)

159	Where residents require lifting at least two members of staff should be on duty at all times.	5.4.2 (51)
160	Where married couples are employed, rotas should allow for shared time off.	5.4.2 (51)
161	Night staff should be experienced and trained. Where night staff are insufficiently experienced it is necessary for senior staff to be on call on the premises.	5.5 (52)
162	The potential therapeutic role of ancillary staff should be recognised.	5.6 (52)
163	Staff involved in meal planning and preparation should receive appropriate training.	5.6.1 (52)
164	Residents' clothing should be well treated, and laundering and needlework should be done with care, whether staff or residents carry out these tasks.	5.6.2 (52)
165	Good maintenance of the building and garden is important for the comfort of residents and should not be neglected.	5.6.4 (53)
166	Clerical staff should be employed to ensure that records and administration are kept up to date without using senior management time inappropriately.	5.6.5 (53)
167	Proprietors should demonstrate that they have considered the range of specialist services residents may require.	5.7 (53)
168	Where specialists are not available through statutory agencies, proprietors must show how such services will be provided and how the costs will be met.	5.7 (53)
169	Management structure should allow for senior staff to be effectively deployed and available at all times.	5.8 (53)
170	Staff induction and training and individual supervision should be carefully considered and planned in detail.	5.8 (53)
171	Proprietors should demonstrate that they are able to provide support for staff to the degree required by the complexity and stress involved in the work, and to enable, through supervision, maximum career development.	5.8 (53)
172	The responsible person in day-to-day charge should have at least one year's experience at senior level in a residential home and/ or a qualification recognised by the registration authority as appropriate for the stated aim of the home.	5.9 (54)
173	The proprietor or responsible person in charge should be able to demonstrate an ability to administer and manage the home on a successful business level.	5.9 (54)
174	Staff deployment should allow for, and the registration authority assist in, the provision of 'in-house' training.	5.9 (54)
175	Staff should be encouraged to undertake appropriate further training.	5.9 (54)

176	The cost of training should be considered when the level of residents' fees is assessed.	5.9 (54)
177	Voluntary workers should be aware of the aims and objectives of the home.	5.10 (54)
178	The role of voluntary workers should be clearly described.	5.10 (54)
179	Staff should be made aware of the expected contribution of voluntary workers.	5.10 (54)

Responsibilities of registration authorities

180	The registration authority should ensure that the care given in the home matches the stated objectives.	6.1 (55)
181	The officer responsible for registration should have experience and ability commensurate with the responsibilities of the job. Other departmental duties should be kept to a minimum.	6.1 (55)
182	The registration authority should provide written guidance on legislation and local conditions to initial enquirers.	6.2 (55)
183	Prospective proprietors should receive counselling and advice on the financial implications and responsibilities of residential care homes.	6.3 (57)
184	The registration authority policy on sponsorship of residents should be explained.	6.3 (57)
185	Prospective proprietors should be informed of the role and responsibilities of other statutory services/ agencies.	6.3 (57)
186	The responsibility of residents in connection with their own financial affairs should be clarified.	6.3 (57)
187	A prospective proprietor should demonstrate to the registration authority competence and understanding in business matters.	6.4 (57)
188	The registration authority should ensure that a check is made on the DHSS list of former proprietors who have been de-registered, before granting registration.	6.4 (57)
189	Registration authorities should consider setting up, in conjunction with other agencies, introduction courses to assist prospective proprietors prepare for this task.	6.4 (57)
190	Registration authorities should ensure that actual and legal divisions of responsibility in voluntary organisations are clearly defined.	6.4 (57)
191	It should be recognised that management bodies may need professional advice on training, costings and staff appointments.	6.4 (57)
192	Progress and preparation for opening a new home should be monitored by the registration authority.	6.5 (58)

193	The need for advice in the early stages should be recognised, to ensure that registration requirements are understood and implemented.	6.5	(58)
194	When residents are placed by social services departments the role of the social worker should be explained.	6.5	(58)
195	Care should be given to explaining the needs of special client groups and those who may be subject to additional legal requirements.	6.5	(58)
196	Information on available community specialist services should be provided to proprietors.	6.5	(58)
197	Managers and staff of homes should have access to training opportunities in the public sector.	6.6	(58)
198	Registration authorities should provide information on alternative training resources.	6.6	(58)
199	Prospective proprietors/ managers should be reminded that they may not operate until a certificate of registration is issued. They should be informed of the penalties for operating un-registered homes.	6.7	(59)
200	Registration authorities should issue certificates of registration as soon as is practicable.	6.7	(59)
201	Proprietors should inform the registration authority of any intended change of ownership.	6.8	(59)
202	Residents should be fully informed of any proposed changes of ownership.	6.8	(59)
203	The registration authority must be informed of any proposed change of objectives or facilities. Such changes must be mutually agreed for the registration to remain valid.	6.9	(59)
204	The brochure should be altered when changes in objectives or facilities are agreed.	6.9	(59)
205	The registration authority should ensure that a visit of inspection is made within three months of registration or where a new manager of a home has been appointed.	6.11	(59)
206	Registration authorities are required by law to inspect homes not less than once every 12 months. It is advised that visits take place more frequently.	6.11	(59)
207	Inspections should focus on the quality of life and care of the residents and on the standards of management.	6.11	(59)
208	A check list should be used as an aid in the formal annual inspection (see Annexe 3 Model 2) but discussion with the proprietor or person in day-to-day charge is also essential.	6.11	(59)
209	The officer making the inspection should identify any change of circumstance which might affect the registration.	6.11	(59)
210	Following the annual review, a written report should be sent to the proprietor.	6.11	(59)

211	Residents should have access freely and in private to the inspection officer when the inspection is made.	6.11 (59)
212	Residents must be told on or before admission how to make complaints to the registered person and to the registration authority.	6.12 (60)
213	Complaints not resolved in the home should be referred to the registration authority in writing for investigation by the authority.	6.12 (60)
214	The registration authority should arrange to interview all persons relevant to the complaint and state in writing to the proprietor, manager and resident the outcome of the investigation, specifying action to be taken.	6.12 (60)
215	Where a registration authority is considering de-registering a home, the proprietor should be informed prior to action being taken.	6.13 (61)
216	Residents, sponsoring agencies and key supporters should be informed that the registration authority intends to take action to de-register the home.	6.13 (61)
217	Registration authorities must make available for inspection at all reasonable times the registers of residential care homes within their area.	6.14 (61)
218	Registration authorities should consider providing general advice on financial assistance for residents and also clarify differences between private and voluntary homes and residential care homes and nursing homes.	6.14 (61)

Annexe 1 References to relevant legislation

Introduction

The legislation quoted below applies in England and Wales. Reference is made specifically to legislation governing the establishment and running of homes, but it should be noted that not all the legislation applies with equal force to all types of establishment; for example, independent schools and housing association projects.

Law and guidance

Acts of Parliament, together with Statutory Instruments, which are Regulations and Orders, are legally binding. In general, observance is the responsibility of local authorities, subject to appeal to the Courts or where appropriate a Tribunal.

'Circulars' come from central government and their purpose is to explain the powers and duties of authorities and to offer helpful guidance. From time to time, draft circulars are subject to a period of discussion, and during this time the guidance contained therein may be followed informally.

Residential care homes registration

Registered Homes Act 1984

This Act governs registration of residential care homes, i.e. any establishment which provides or is intended to provide, whether for reward or not, residential accommodation with both board and personal care for four or more persons in need of personal care by reason of old age, disablement, past or present dependence on alcohol or drugs, or past or present mental disorder.

Regulations

Regulations to be issued towards the end of 1984 will specify in detail requirements concerning the conduct of residential care homes.

Circulars

A circular will provide guidance on the above regulations and arrangements.

Another circular on nursing homes will provide guidance on regulations relevant to dually registered homes.

Fire precautions

Draft guide to fire precautions in existing residential care premises

In most residential care homes, control over fire safety is exercised through the statutory provisions relating to registration. However, in certain cases, other statutory provisions may apply and there could be overlap between the legislation. (This is explained in DHSS circular LAC(83)4, Welsh Office circular 9/83.) It is for the appropriate authorities to decide which statutory provisions should apply in any particular case. In considering the appropriate fire safety standards for such premises, the fire authority will normally have regard to the recommendations in the Home Office *Draft guide to fire precautions in existing residential care premises*, which was issued in January 1983 (LAC(83)4, Welsh Office circular 9/84). For registration purposes, the local social services authority will want to be satisfied that the fire authority's recommendations have been met.

Building Regulations (SI 1976 No.1676) and amendments

The requirements for structural fire safety in the Regulations apply to the construction of new buildings and to alterations, extensions and changes of use in England and Wales, except in Inner London where separate building bye-laws apply. 'Purpose groups' are defined to clarify different types of buildings and specify the technical requirements of the Regulations which apply for safety purposes. Institutional uses include hospitals, homes, schools or other similar establishments used as living accommodation for, or for the treatment, care or maintenance of persons suffering from disabilities due to old age, illness, or other physical or mental disability or under the age of five years where people sleep on the premises (Purpose Group 2).

The other relevant purpose group involves accommodation for residential purposes other than any of those listed above, and here different standards will apply (Purpose Group 3).

District Councils administer and enforce the Building Regulations.

Welfare

Mental Health Act 1983

Section 115 empowers local authority mental welfare officers to enter and inspect any premises where a mentally disordered person is living, if there is reason to believe he is not under proper care. DHSS circular LAC(83)7, Welsh Office circular 36/83 explained that mental welfare officers are to be replaced by approved social workers from 28 October 1984.

Circulars

Ministry of Health and Welsh Board of Health Circular 18/60 (paragraphs 34 and 35) and paragraphs 248 and 249 of the Memorandum enclosed with Circular 17/60, explain the circumstances under which a mental welfare officer may enter and inspect premises under section 22 of the *Mental Health Act 1959* (see above). Obstruction of him by a householder is not an offence under the Act, unless a mentally disordered person is living on the premises and there was reasonable cause to believe he was not under proper care. The consent of the householder to enter is necessary unless, exceptionally, a justice's warrant—addressed to a constable—has been obtained.

Ministry of Health and Welsh Board of Health Circular 22/65, *National Assistance Act 1948; Welfare of Handicapped Persons*, includes advice on residential accommodation for the physically handicapped.

Health Services and Public Health Act 1968 and DHSS Circular 19/71, Welsh Office circular 47/71, *Welfare of the Elderly,* deals with authorities' powers to provide *inter alia.* assistance in finding suitable households for boarding elderly persons, visiting and advisory services and social work support; and recreation facilities.

DHSS circular LAC 13/74, Welsh Office circular 46/74, includes local authority sponsorship of elderly and disabled residents in voluntary homes and those registered under the *Registered Homes Act 1984* and authorities' powers to assist the disabled to find suitable supportive lodgings.

DHSS circular LAC 19/74, Welsh Office circular 100/74, gives general approval to local authorities to provide a range of residential accommodation for the mentally disordered whether in premises managed by the Council or otherwise, on such conditions as may be agreed. This wide approval would include placements in private or voluntary homes or boarding out in private households, whether or not the premises are registered under the *Registered Homes Act 1984.*

DHSS circular HN(80)35, WHN(81)4, draws attention to the National Development Group for the Mentally Handicapped, *Improving the quality of services for mentally handicapped people: a check list of standards.* It consists of a series of questions each of which implies a standard.

Planning and building

Town and Country Planning Act 1971

This Act requires planning permission to be obtained for any material change in the use of buildings or land. *The Town and Country Planning (Use Classes) Order* (SI 1385/72) provides that changes of use between uses falling within Class XIV do not require planning permission; Class XIV includes use as a home or institution providing for the boarding, care and maintenance of children, old people or persons under disability; a convalescent home; a nursing home; a sanatorium; or a hospital.

Housing Association hostels

Standards in this accommodation are governed by the Housing Corporation's design and contract criteria for shared housing.

Independent schools

Standards in independent schools approved by the Secretary of State for Education and Science or the Secretary of State for Wales under the *Education Act 1981* are required to conform, so far as is practicable, to the *Education (School Premises) Regulations 1981* (SI 909/1981). It would be relevant to have regard to these standards in determining those for other independent schools that fall to be registered as residential care homes.

Building notes	*Local Authority Building Note No. 2* provides guidelines for residential accommodation for elderly people (under revision).
	Local Authority Building Note No. 8 covers residential accommodation for mentally handicapped adults.
Circulars	DHSS circular LASSL 75 (19) gives the Department's recommendations on residential accommodation for physically handicapped people. DHSS circular LASSL 78(6) gives the maximum recommended areas for residential and other accommodation.

Staff employment

Rehabilitation of Offenders Act 1974 (Exceptions) Order 1975 (SI 1023/1975)	Under the *Rehabilitation of Offenders Act 1974* a person who received a non-custodial sentence, or a custodial sentence of not more than 30 months, and is not reconvicted during a specified period, becomes a rehabilitated person. His conviction then becomes 'spent', i.e. it is regarded in law for most purposes as never having occurred. The effect of this is that the person applying for work is entitled to deny that he has ever been convicted; and the employer, if he somehow learns of the spent conviction, is not entitled to refuse to employ him, dismiss him or prejudice him in any other way because of it.

There are, however, certain types of employment (listed in the 1975 Order) where this does not apply, provided that when asked about previous convictions, the person is told that by virtue of the Order spent convictions must be declared. The exceptions include:

Occupations concerned with carrying on an establishment required to be registered under the *Registered Homes Act 1984*. Any employment by a local authority in connection with the provision of social services, which would enable the person concerned to have access in the course of his normal duties to certain classes of person. These include people aged over 65, children, those suffering from mental disorders and those who are seriously disabled. (This applies to employment both in premises registered under the *Registered Homes Act 1984* and those not so registered.)

Professions Supplementary to Medicine Regulations 1964 and 1968	The *National Assistance (Professions Supplementary to Medicine) Regulations 1964* (SI 939/ 1964), as amended by the *National Assistance (Professions Supplementary to Medicine) (Amendment) Regulations 1968* (SI 271/ 1968) prohibit the employment by a voluntary organisation for the purposes of providing services under Part III of the *National Assistance Act 1948* of chiropodists, dietitians, occupational therapists, physiotherapists, remedial gymnasts or orthoptists unless they are registered under the *Professions Supplementary to Medicine Act 1960*.

Catering and health

Catering in homes for elderly people

This 1975 booklet deals with suitable types of food, menu planning, budgeting, purchasing and storage, preparation, hygiene and serving. The booklet is in need of some revision; copies can be obtained from the Catering and Dietetics Division, Department of Health and Social Security, Alexander Fleming House, London SE1, or from Catering Adviser, Welsh Office, Cathays Park, Cardiff CF1 3NQ.

Arrangements for health care

DHSS/Welsh Office memorandum *Residential homes for the elderly: arrangements for health care (1977)* (DHSS circular HC(77)25, LAC (77)13 and Welsh Office circular 117/77, WHC(77)30) gives guidance on the availability to residents of community health services. This guidance is also applicable to other residential care homes.

Taxes

Finance Act 1972

Schedule 5, Group 7, item 4, exempts for Value Added Tax charges for care in old people's homes and homes for the disabled and mentally disordered registered under the *Registered Homes Act 1984.*

Race relations

Race Relations Act 1976 (Sections 20 and 22(2)(b)) and Racial discrimination: a guide to the Race Relations Act 1975

It is unlawful for anyone providing accommodation to the public, or a section of the public, in a hotel, boarding house or other similar establishment, or the services of any trade or business, to discriminate directly or indirectly against a person on racial grounds (colour, race, nationality or ethnic or national origins). Premises are exempt from the Act if the proprietor, or his near relative (wife or husband, parent or child, grandparent or grandchild, or brother or sister), lives and intends to continue to live on the premises and shares accommodation (other than storage accommodation or means of access) with other persons living there who are not members of his household, and the residential accommodation is not normally provided there for more than six persons.

Health and safety at work

The Health and Safety at Work Act 1974.

Education

Education Act 1981.

Annexe 2 Relevant organisations

The following list gives names and brief details of organisations which provide training, advice or useful publications. Most of them are not involved with giving direct care although a few do run residential care homes. It is not possible to include here all relevant agencies; details of these will be available from the National Council for Voluntary Organisations, (NCVO) 26 Bedford Square, London, WC1 (01-636 4066) or from the Wales Council for Voluntary Action, Llys Ifor, Crescent Road, Caerphilly CF8 1XL (0222 869224).

People with physical and sensory handicaps

British Association of the Hard of Hearing
7–11 Armstrong Road, London, W3 01-743 1110

Aims
To deal with all problems arising from impaired hearing: to act as an information and advice centre; to assist in the development of government services for the hard of hearing; to foster social and cultural activities; to co-operate with organisations throughout the world which have similar objects.

Activities
The development of clubs and classes throughout the country; co-operation with relevant government departments and other voluntary organisations; organisation of educational and recreational activities; advice on hearing aid problems; help with vocational problems; encouragement of the practice of lip-reading and improvement of speech.

British Deaf Association
38 Victoria Place, Carlisle, Cumbria CA1 1HU 0228-48844

Aims
The Association is concerned with the interests, problems and needs of all deaf people, particularly those most profoundly affected by deafness—those who were born deaf and those who were deafened early in life.

Activities
Problems of the deaf in education, employment and social services are studied and information made available to interested authorities on the experience of people suffering the difficulties of their own lifelong deafness. The Association makes special provision for summer schools, school leaver courses and family summer schools. Community holidays for elderly deaf people are arranged where their own special needs are catered for.

Centre on Environment for the Handicapped
126 Albert Street, London, NW1 7NF 01-482 2247

Aims
To help handicapped people by making architects and other professionals better informed about special needs and the ways in which buildings and other facilities can best serve them.

Activities	Architectural consultancy service; information servic multi-disciplinary seminars; library.
Publications	List available.

Chest, Heart and Stroke Association
Tavistock House North, Tavistock Square,
London WC1H 9JE 01-387 3012

Aims	To work for the prevention of chest, heart and stroke i nesses, and to help people who suffer from them.
Activities	A continuing programme of research, health educatio rehabilitation, welfare and counselling services. The Assoc ation also publishes books, posters and leaflets, and orga ises conferences.

Disability Alliance
25 Denmark Street, London, WC2 8NJ 01-240 0806

Aims	To persuade society to pay an income as of right and c equitable principles to all disabled persons, according to tt severity of their disability.
Activities	The Alliance is a federation of over 50 organisations of ar for disabled people who have joined together to press f a comprehensive income scheme on a common platforr The Alliance gives information and advice on welfare righ queries; holds conferences and runs campaigns on topic issues; publishes a series of research pamphlets on tt financial consequences of disablement; supports loc advisory projects for disabled people; and comments c proposed and existing legislation.
Publications	List available.

Disabled Living Foundation
346 Kensington High Street, London W14 8NS
01-602 2491

Aims	The terms of reference include all disabilities (mental, phys cal, and sensory) together with multiple handicaps and tt infirmities of age. The Foundation works on those aspec of ordinary life which present special problems and diff culties to disabled people of all ages and disabilities. Pure medical matters are excluded.
Activities	An information service collects, stores and distribute information concerning disability to all those concerne with disabled people, both personally and professionall the incontinence advisory service gives information ar guidance in response to enquiries from those affected t incontinence, their families and those concerned pr fessionally; the clothing advisory service gives help ar guidance concerning clothing enquiries; the aids centre a standing exhibition of aids and equipment designed reduce the effects of residual disability. The main purpos

is to provide practical information and demonstration to all those professionally concerned, but disabled people and/ or their relatives are also welcome.

Publications   List available.

Disablement Information Advice Line (DIAL)
DIAL House, 117 High Street, Clay Cross, Chesterfield, Derbyshire S45 9DZ 0246 864498

Aims and
Activities   To provide a free, impartial and confidential service of information, advice and, in some cases, practical help for disabled people, supplied by people with direct personal experience of disability.

Leukaemia Society
Hamlyns View, St Andrew's Road, Exeter EX1 2AF

Aims   To promote the welfare of people suffering from leukaemia and that of their families, and also the welfare of those families who have lost relatives from the disease.

Activities   The Society provides information, support, financial help and holidays.

**National Association for Deaf-Blind and
Rubella Handicapped (SENSE Association)**
311 Grays Inn Road, London WC1X 8PT 01-278 1000

Aims   To provide information and guidance to parents and professionals working with deaf-blind children and young adults.

Activities   Has information and advisory service. Runs parents' groups and staff seminars. Has a residential Centre, a school and organises holiday facilities. Local groups.

Publications   List available.

Multiple Sclerosis Society of Great Britain and Northern Ireland
286 Munster Road, London SW6 6AP 01-381 4022

Aims   To promote and fund medical research. To provide a welfare and support service for families, one member of whom suffers from multiple sclerosis.

Activities   A comprehensive welfare and support service through a network of 350 branches and associations. Holiday and short-stay homes. Fund-raising for research.

Parkinson's Disease Society
36 Portland Place, London W1N 3DG 01-323 1174

Aims   To help patients and their relatives with problems in the home arising from Parkinson's Disease; to collect and disseminate information on the disease; to encourage and provide funds for research into the disease; to publish helpful literature; to establish branches.

Royal Association for Disability and Rehabilitation (RADAR)
25 Mortimer Street, London W1N 8AB 01-637 5400

Aims

To improve the environment for disabled people.

Activities

RADAR is a co-ordinating body with nearly 400 member associations. It acts as a pressure group on central and local government and has an active legal and parliamentary committee which liaises closely with the All-Party Disablement Group. RADAR is concerned with every aspect of disability but is particularly involved with access, education, employment, holidays, housing, mobility and welfare. Rehabilitation Engineering Advisory Panels, comprising groups of voluntary engineers, with the help of therapists, devise mobility aids which are not available commercially. A publications department issues a comprehensive range of books, pamphlets, etc. List available.

Royal Association in Aid of the Deaf and Dumb
27 Old Oak Road, London W3 7AN 01-743 6187

Aims

To promote the spiritual, social and general welfare of deaf people so that they may develop their full potential.

Activities

The Association works primarily with people of all ages who have a hearing impediment from birth or early childhood and offers help to those with additional handicaps. Trained staff act as interpreters and advise and help with everyday problems; special services include churches, social clubs and recreational facilities, and work in hospitals.

Royal National Institute for the Blind
224 Great Portland Street, London W1N 6AA
01-388 1266

Aims

To promote the better education, training, employment and welfare of blind people, and generally to watch over their interests and to further the prevention of blindness.

Activities

Production of braille books, periodicals and music. Moon books and periodicals; students' braille and tape libraries talking book library; sale of aids and equipment at subsidised prices; education advisory service, nursery and other schools for blind and additionally handicapped children homes, hostels and holiday hotels; rehabilitation centres for people who have lost their sight; school of physiotherapy commercial college for blind switchboard operators, shorthand and audio-typists and computer programmers; vocational assessment centre for school leavers; home worker scheme; employment service; reference library of printed works on blindness.

Publications

List available.

Royal National Institute for the Deaf
105 Gower Street, London WC1E 6AH 01-387 8033

Aims
To protect and promote the interests and well-being of all deaf people in the United Kingdom.

Activities
The institute encourages research into the prevention and mitigation of deafness, and works to improve conditions affecting the education, employment and general welfare of those who are deaf. Special residential services for deaf and deaf/blind people, including rehabilitation and training programmes, as well as longer-term home care. Supportive hostel accommodation in London providing a link to employment, and a technical trainee centre. Scientific and technical departments in London and Glasgow advise on a variety of devices. The Social Services Department helps those who contact RNID about social difficulties. The library is one of the foremost in the world on speech and hearing disorders.

The Spastics Society
12 Park Crescent, London W1N 4EQ 01-636 5020

Aims and Activities
The world's leading organisation in the field of cerebral palsy. It promotes facilities for the treatment, education and training of spastic children and adults. It is sponsoring paediatric and educational research programmes and, in co-operation with its local groups, maintains over 160 schools and centres of various kinds.

SPOD
(Sexual and Personal Relationships of the Disabled)
286 Camden Road, London N7 0BJ 01-607 8851

Aims
To provide information and advice on sexual, personal and emotional problems which disability can cause.

Activities
Runs information and advisory service for both consumers and professionals working with them. Can arrange counselling. Produces teaching materials and runs training courses.

Publications
List available.

People with mental handicap and mentally ill people

Advocacy Alliance
115 Golden Lane, London EC1Y 0TJ 01-253 2056

Aims
To ensure that mentally handicapped people in long-stay hospitals receive all the help, benefits and advice they are entitled to.

Activities
To supply independent advocates on a one-to-one basis to represent mentally handicapped people in long-stay hospitals.

Publications
List available.

Alzheimer's Disease Society
3rd Floor, Bank Building, Fulham Broadway,
London SW6 1EP 01-381 3177

Aims	To give support to families; to disseminate knowledge of the illness and aids available; to try and ensure adequate nursing care; to promote research and public education through press, media and fund-raising.
Activities	Forming local branches for relatives of patients; informing health and social workers and pressing for improved facilities locally; raising funds to support hospices, day centres and research.

Association of Professions for the Mentally Handicapped
Kings Fund Centre, 126 Albert Street, London, NW1 7NF
01-267 6111

Aims	To promote the general welfare of mentally handicapped people and their families by encouraging high standards of care and development for mentally handicapped people and by facilitating the sharing of knowledge and collaboration between professionals working in this field.
Activities	Local groups and divisions. Runs regular seminars and courses and publishes newsletter.
Publications	List available.

Association of Residential Communities for the Mentally Retarded
PO Box 4, Lydney, Gloucestershire 0594 530 398

Aims	To encourage good practice concerning the assessment and review of residents in centres for the mentally handicapped, and to provide a multiplicity of services of the very highest order.
Activities	It monitors standards of care and publishes advisory pamphlets and issues information on all aspects of the care of the mentally handicapped. Its membership is open to anyone and any organisation which is involved in the care of such people.
Publications	List available.

British Institute for Mental Handicap
Wolverhampton Road, Kidderminster, Worcs DY10 3PP
0562 850251

Aims	To raise the standards of current services and provision for mentally handicapped people and those professionally involved with them in the community and NHS settings.
Activities	Library and information service. Regular Bulletin, together with conferences and seminars run on regional basis. Runs current awareness service which lists new publications and initiatives in the mental handicap field.
Publications	List available.

Campaign for Mentally Handicapped People
12A Maddox Street, London W1R 9PL 01-492 0727

Aims
To work for the rights of mentally handicapped people; to ensure that their pattern and conditions of life are as close as possible to those of non-handicapped people, and that they participate in decisions which affect their lives.

Activities
Contact with central and local government and health authorities; collection and dissemination of information on current services and new ideas; publication of discussion and research papers.

Publications
List available.

Independent Development Council for People with Mental Handicap
Kings Fund Centre, 126 Albert Street, London NW1 7NF 01-267 6111

Aims
To promote nationally the development of appropriate services for people with mental handicap and their families.

Activities
The Council offers advice on good practice and the local action necessary to introduce and sustain better services for mentally handicapped people. It aims to offer strategic advice to relevant agencies and individuals on the development of community-based services and the effective implementation of new policies in the mental handicap field.

Publications
List available.

MIND (National Association for Mental Health)
22 Harley Street, London W1N 2ED 01-637 0741

Aims
To promote mental health and help the mentally disordered; to press for improvements in the statutory mental health services; to promote research; to help the work of nearly 200 local mental health associations throughout the country.

Activities
Conferences and short courses on a wide range of mental health issues, exploring new concepts. Other short courses for teachers, doctors, clergy, social workers, residential and day care workers, and nurses. Advisory casework service staffed by trained social workers. Pilot projects in community services; educational campaigns. Legal and welfare rights service to protect the rights of patients and mental health workers and to iron out anomalies in the law. A lawyers' group brings test cases on selected issues involving mental health and child care legislation.

Richmond Fellowship
8 Addison Road, London W14 8DL 01-603 6373

Aims
To provide residential accommodation in the form of therapeutic communities for the rehabilitation of those who are or have been emotionally or mentally disturbed or who are

87

at risk, and for those who are overcoming a problem involving drug or alcohol abuse; to educate the general public in the functions of such half-way houses, particularly through involvement in the Fellowship's work.

Activities Runs 37 therapeutic communities, both short and long stay, catering for a variety of diagnostic and age groups. Provides through its own college a comprehensive programme of education in mental health, human relations, pastoral care, group work, counselling and residential social work.

Royal Society for Mentally Handicapped Children and Adults
Mencap National Centre, 123 Golden Lane,
London EC1Y 0RT 01-253 9433

Aims To secure for mentally handicapped people provision commensurate with their needs. To increase public awareness of the problems faced by mentally handicapped people and their families.

Activities Offers support for parents of mentally handicapped children through its network of 450 local societies and twelve regional offices. Finances research into causation of mental handicap; provides specialist information and advisory services for lay people and professional workers. Holds symposia and conferences. Continued education and work training schemes unit at Westhill College, Birmingham. Leisure facilities through the National Federation of Gateway Clubs. Publicity material and films available.

Publications List available.

Children and young people

Child Poverty Action Group
1 Macklin Street, London WC2B 5NH
01-242 3225/ 9149

Aims To promote action for the relief directly or indirectly of poverty among children and families with children.

Activities Research into and publication of facts regarding family poverty in Britain. Investigation of methods of preventing poverty—e.g. child benefits and other social benefits. Providing information on existing benefits, including the use of appeal machinery, to social workers, trade unionists and others.

Children's Legal Centre
20 Compton Terrace, London N1 2UN 01-359 9392

Aims To represent the interests of children and young people in matters of law and policy affecting them.

Activities Free advice and information service by letter and telephone (2 to 5 p.m. weekdays). Monitoring and making representations on law and policy. Taking test cases. Publishing, education and training.

| Publications | List available. |

Invalid Children's Aid Association
126 Buckingham Palace Road, London SW1W 9SB
01-730 9891

Aims	To help handicapped children and their families to live as full a life as possible regardless of the type of handicap.
Activities	Provides free help and advice for parents with handicapped children. An information service deals with general enquiries; the secretary for schools will advise on educational problems; a social work service operates in London and some of the home counties. ICAA runs five residential schools; two for severely asthmatic boys and three for children with speech and language disorders. Publications on relevant subjects with particular emphasis on speech and language disorders.
Publications	List available.

National Association of Young People in Care (NAYPIC)
Salem House, 28A Manor Row, Bradford BD1 4QU
0274 728484/733134

| Aims | To improve conditions of young people in care and after care; to promote the views and opinions of young people in care; and wherever possible to help start, support and develop local groups. |
| Activities | Advice and help by letter and telephone; support for local groups; social events. |

National Association of Young People's Counselling and Advisory Services
National Youth Bureau, 17–23 Albion Street,
Leicester LE1 6GD 0533 554775

Aims	To bring together services and individuals from a wide range of young people's counselling and advisory services and befriending projects.
Activities	Information on counselling services (with extensive local contacts). Development Officer in association with the National Youth Bureau can advise on the development of new services. Can provide support and training.
Publications	List available.

National Children's Bureau
8 Wakley Street, Islington, London EC1V 7QE
01-278 9441

| Aims | A national inter-disciplinary organisation concerned with children's needs in the family, school and society. It achieves its objects through a membership composed of local authorities, professional associations, voluntary |

bodies, universities and other educational institutions and individuals.

Activities Research into normal child development from educational, social, psychological and medical aspects, as well as children with special needs. There are local groups of the Bureau in different parts of the country. Information and library service available to enquirers in office hours.

Publications List available.

National Council of Voluntary Child Care Organisations
40 Brunswick Square, London WC1N 1AU 01-837 2221

Aims The relief of necessitous children and the furtherance and protection of the common interest of children in the care of voluntary organisations.

Activities Maintaining a link between the member organisations and voluntary and statutory agencies, especially the Department of Health and Social Security, the local authorities and the Central Council for Education and Training in Social Work. Advising and representing member organisations at their request. Membership is open to voluntary organisations engaged in social work for necessitous children.

National Deaf Children's Society
45 Hereford Road, London, W2 5AH 01-229 9272/4

Aims To obtain for deaf children the best possible medical, audiological, educational and welfare services; to support their families and to inform the general public about childhood deafness.

Activities Free advice and information service on all aspects of childhood deafness; nationwide home assistant scheme; organises courses and conferences; provides holidays, welfare grants, hearing aids and other equipment. 140 registered groups represent the needs of deaf children both locally and nationally.

Publications List available.

National Autistic Society
276 Willesden Lane, London NW2 5RB 01-451 3844

Aims To provide and promote day and residential centres for the care and education of autistic children and for those who were autistic as children. To help parents, particularly by arranging meetings. To encourage research. To stimulate more understanding between doctors, teachers and the general public.

Activities The Society runs an advisory and information service for parents and professionally interested people on the nature of childhood autism, the type of service needed and teaching methods; publishes and distributes literature on the management and education of autistic children; runs schools and adult centres. Local affiliated societies also run schools and adult centres. Conferences held twice yearly.

Publications List available.

National Society for the Prevention of Cruelty to Children (NSPCC)
67 Saffron Hill, London EC1 01-242 1626

Aims To prevent child abuse in all forms; to give practical help to families and children at risk; to encourage greater public awareness and understanding of the problem; to initiate research and new methods of treatment.

Activities NSPCC Special Units offer professional advice and consultation to other agencies. The Society maintains a network of over 60 therapeutic play groups. Its School of Social Work offers training to its own and other professional staff.

Publications List available.

National Youth Bureau
17–23 Albion Street, Leicester, LE1 6GD 0533 554 775

Aims To provide a forum and national resource agency for the wide range of practitioners (both professional and voluntary) who are concerned with youth affairs and the social education of young people.

Activities Information, training and research services. Free enquiry service based on extensive collection of documents relating to young people. Various research projects. Publication of journals, books, reports.

Publications List available.

Voluntary Council for Handicapped Children
8 Wakley Street, London EC1V 7QE 01-278 9441

Aims An independently elected Council, providing an inter-disciplinary forum for statutory, professional and voluntary organisations with an interest in services for disabled children and young people.

Activities Free advice and information service on all aspects of disability, including current developments in health, education and social services. Has extensive contacts with local and national voluntary organisations and runs regular seminars, study days and training programmes.

Publications List available.

Elderly people

Age Concern England (National Old People's Welfare Council)
60 Pitcairn Road, Mitcham, Surrey CR4 3LL 01-640 5431

Aims To promote the welfare of elderly people, through training, media information and advice, and of workers with or for the elderly.

Activities	Acts as a centre of information, policy, research and social advocacy on subjects pertaining to the welfare of elderly people and makes representations on their behalf. Over 1,300 local Age Concern/Old People's Welfare groups provide a range of practical services.
Publications	List available.

British Association for Service to the Elderly (BASE)
3 Keele Farm House, Keele, Staffs ST5 5HA
0782 627280

Aims	To improve the health and welfare of the elderly, to achieve this mainly through the medium of education and dissemination of authoritative information concerning the problems elderly people face today, with practical guidance about ways of tackling these. BASE is committed to the notion that care should be enabling rather than disabling. BASE is fully multi-disciplinary/inter-disciplinary and anyone in sympathy with its aims may join.

Centre for Policy on Ageing
(formerly National Corporation for the Care of Old People)
Nuffield Lodge Studio, Regent's Park, London NW1 4RS
01-586 9844/9

Aims	To encourage better services for elderly people by promoting informed debate, stimulating awareness of the needs of older people, formulating and promoting policies and encouraging the spread of good practice.
Activities	Policy studies undertaken on a variety of subjects, e.g. services for the mentally ill, education, transport, civil liberties. Library and information service for those professionally interested.
Publications	*New literature on old age* (bi-monthly). Directory of research. Various reports. List available.

Christian Council on Ageing
Greens Norton Court, Greens Norton, Nr. Towcester,
Northants NN12 8BS 0327 50481

Aims and Activities	The Council is concerned with the life of the spirit, as well as with mind and body. In seeking to assist men and women to find fullness of life, it has the active elderly in mind as well as the handicapped and frail. This is where faith comes in, and the appreciation so often given to those who offer pastoral care gives overwhelming evidence of its importance. This is an aspect of the Council's work that complements what others are doing, and it is hoped that its significance will be widely recognised.

Counsel and Care for the Elderly (Elderly Invalids Fund)
131 Middlesex Street, London E1 7JF 01-621 1624

Aims
To provide an advice and counselling service to pensioners on any matters which concern them. To make provision for nursing home care when needed. To give financial help where needed towards nursing home fees or home equipment.

Activities
Trained caseworkers deal with enquiries from pensioners, their relatives and friends, health authorities and social services, mainly concerning accommodation and financial assistance.

Help the Aged
St James' Walk, London EC1R 0BE 01-253 0253

Aims
An international organisation which aims to relieve the distress of the world's aged. The long-term aim is to provide or arrange conditions whereby the elderly may live their lives to the full as integrated members of society until the end of their days.

Activities
Day centres and work centres; minibuses and mobile chiropody units. Campaigns for better pensions system and flexible retirement age.

National Council for Carers and their Elderly Dependants
29 Chilworth Mews, London W2 3RG 01-262 1451

Aims
To help single people who have or have had the care of elderly or infirm dependants.

Activities
The Council gives advisory service by correspondence; campaigns for increased social security benefits and for wider domiciliary services; promotes holiday relief and sitter-in help; organises conferences; runs penfriends club. As a housing society it intends to set up sheltered housing for single people who go out to work leaving an elderly relative at home. It has some forty branches throughout the United Kingdom.

People recovering from drug addiction and alcohol abuse

Alcoholics Anonymous
11 Redcliffe Gardens, London SW10 9BQ

General Services Office UK 01-352 9779
London Enquiries 01-834 8202

Aims
A fellowship of men and women who share their experience, strength and hope with each other that they may solve their common problem and help others to recover from alcoholism. The only requirement for membership is an honest desire to stop drinking. AA has no dues or fees. The primary purpose is to stay sober and help other alcoholics to achieve sobriety.

Activities	Over 1,500 groups in the United Kingdom.
Publications	List available.

Alcohol Concern
(The National Agency on Alcohol Abuse)
3 Grosvenor Crescent, London, SW1 6LO 01-235 4182

Aims and Activities	Set up in 1983 to promote services for people suffering from drink-related problems; help the prevention of such problems; advance the education of the public about the effect on society of the abuse of alcohol; and to improve the provision of education for paid or volunteer professionals working with problem drinkers. Grant-aided by the DHSS. Membership open to individuals and organisations.

Institute for the Study of Drug Dependence
Kingsbury House, 3 Blackburn Road, London NW6 1XA
01-328 5541/2

Aims and Activities	An independent non-profit organisation. Its information service covers all aspects of non-medical use of drugs, backed by a library of over 30,000 articles and books, and is available free to any enquirer. Its Evaluation and Research Unit is engaged in evaluating drug education in schools and developing effective teaching approaches.

National Association for the Care and Resettlement of Offenders (NACRO)
169 Clapham Road, London SW9 0PU 01-582 6500

Aims	To provide national leadership to voluntary bodies involved in the prevention of crime and the care (including the after-care) of offenders; and to involve members of the community in all forms of crime prevention and the resettlement of offenders.
Activities	To pioneer new projects, experiment, initiate research, train hostel staff, service voluntary agencies and co-ordinate their work with that of the statutory and other voluntary social services. Ordinary membership open to bodies active in this field; associate membership open to bodies or individuals who are interested. NACRO has replaced, and taken over, the work of the former National Association of Discharged Prisoners Aid Societies.

Release
1 Elgin Avenue, London W9 01-289 1123
01-603 8654 for 24 hour emergency service.

Aims and Activities	A free service for those in trouble or difficulty, including those arrested, to help them talk freely about their position and problems and obtain further information and help. Legal advice, drugs advice and referrals are all offered. The agency has two full-time counsellors specialising in pregnancy advice. Any age helped.

94

Standing Conference on Drug Abuse (SCODA)
3 Blackburn Road, London NW6 1XA 01-328 6556/7

Activities
The national co-ordinating body for non-statutory services dealing with problems of drug abuse. Organises quarterly general meetings. Produces a 6-weekly newsletter. Apply for details.

General section

Asian Community Action Group
15 Bedford Road, London SW4 01-733 7494

Activities
Runs an advisory service for all client groups in the Asian Community.

British Association of Social Workers
16 Kent Street, Birmingham B5 6RD 021-622 3911

Aims
To promote the sciences and arts which comprise social work and the better education and training of social workers; to provide a professional organisation for and of those engaged in social work and to promote and advance such work, its standards and ideals and to foster public knowledge and appreciation of their work; to provide opportunities for the social work profession to work in unity towards the promotion of welfare of individuals and the social well-being of the community by encouragement of good social work practice.

Membership qualifications
Membership: for professionally qualified social workers/ residential social workers; associateship: for unqualified social workers/ residential social workers; studentship: for students on courses leading to professional qualifications in social work/ residential social work, and trainee social workers. Fees vary according to salary and status.

Publications
Social Work Today, British Journal of Social Work, occasional publications.

Central Council for Education and Training in Social Work (CCETSW)
Derbyshire House, St Chad's Street, London WC1
01-278 2455

Aims
Promotes, develops and validates education and training for social work and care staff in residential, day, domiciliary, field and community services throughout the UK. Courses are validated in universities, polytechnics and colleges of higher and further education. Qualifying courses lead to the Certificate of Qualification in Social Work (CQSW) and the Certificate in Social Service (CSS). Approves post-qualifying studies.

Advises employing agencies about in-service training and staff development. CCETSW-approved In-service Courses in Social Care (ICSC) in local colleges offer day-release training for care staff. Courses leading to the Preliminary Certificate in Social Care (PCSC) introduce young people to a variety of careers in the social services.

Jewish Welfare Board
(Board of Guardians and Trustees
for the Relief of Jewish Poor),
221 Golders Green Road, London NW11 9DW
01-458 3282

Aims
To provide a comprehensive range of social services for the benefit of members of the Jewish community.

Activities
Welfare services and counselling, residential homes for the aged, sheltered housing for the elderly, family housing, psychiatric after-care hostels and day centres, day and community centres for the elderly, careers guidance.

King's Fund Centre
126 Albert Street, London NW1 7NF 01-267 6111

Aims
The Centre is maintained by King Edward's Hospital Fund for London. The aims of the Centre are to provide a forum for discussion and study, and to help accelerate the intro-duction of good ideas and practice in the planning and management of health services.

Activities
To achieve the above aims, conferences and meetings are held, small exhibitions are mounted, and there is an active information service based on the Centre's extensive library.

Publications
List available.

National Federation of Housing Associations
30/32 Southampton Street, Strand, London WC2E 7HE
01-240 2771/7

Aims
To promote housing associations as defined in Section 129 of the Housing Act 1974. To guide and co-ordinate the policy of its existing 2,000 member societies and to represent their interests to government, local authorities and the Housing Corporation.

Activities
Provides liaison particularly with the Department of the Environment and the Registrar of Friendly Societies. Provides advice and common services for its members; arranges training courses and conferences; carries out research and publishes specialist literature; associated with two charitable trusts concerned with housing the elderly.

Publications
Voluntary Housing (monthly), Year Book. List available.

Social Care Association
(formerly Residential Care Association)
23A Victoria Road, Surbiton, Surrey KT6 4JZ
01-390 6831

Aims
To promote and encourage a high standard of service for people receiving care. To promote and maintain a high

standard of training and professional practice in the care services and to promote a wide range of developments in care services.

Westindian Concern Ltd
(in association with Caribbean House Group)
Caribbean House, Bridport Place, Shoreditch Park,
London N1 5DS 01-729 0986

Aims
: To promote the social, educational, spiritual and economic wellbeing of West Indians in the UK and elsewhere.

Activities
: Family casework and pastoral service, community homes with education, supervision and IT day-care provision, job training and courses for those working with West Indians.

Publications
: List available.

There are also local and county associations of registered homes. Registration authorities will have the addresses of local secretaries. Many associations are affiliated to the National Confederation of Registered Rest Homes Associations. At the time of publication the Hon. Secretary is A. F. Andrews, 74 London Road, St. Leonards on Sea, East Sussex TN37 6AS.

Annexe 3 Application for registration
Model 1 form

Suggested model for use by applicants wishing to register homes under the Registered Homes Act 1984

Home for (Please specify number of residents to be accommodated.)

a   Elderly persons

b   Physically handicapped adults

c   Physically handicapped children

d   Mentally handicapped adults

e   Mentally handicapped children

f   Persons recovering from mental illness

g   Persons recovering from alcohol dependency

h   Persons recovering from drug dependency

Name or title of home

Address

Tel. no.

Date to be opened

Brief statement of main aims and objectives of home

Section 1 The Applicants

Particulars of owners of the home

Full name   Mr/ Mrs/ Miss/ Ms   **Date of birth**

Full name   Mr/ Mrs/ Miss/ Ms   **Date of birth**

Address (if other than above)

If Home is to be owned on a partnership basis please give details of partners.

Full name   Mr/ Mrs/ Miss/ Ms   **Date of birth**

Full name   Mr/ Mrs/ Miss/ Ms   **Date of birth**

Full name   Mr/ Mrs/ Miss/ Ms   **Date of birth**

Address

Tel. no.

f application for registration is to be made on behalf of a voluntary organisation or company.

Name of organisation or company _____

Address _____

_____

                              Tel no. _____

Give name and address of the Chairman and Secretary of the Home's Management Committee/ Company and Chairman and Secretary of Board of Directors or like persons.

Name _____

Address _____

_____

_____

Particulars of proposed Manager(s)/ Officer(s) in Charge of the home if other than the owners.

Full name _____ Mr/ Mrs/ Miss/ Ms   **Date of birth** _____

Full name _____ Mr/ Mrs/ Miss/ Ms   **Date of birth** _____

Private address _____

                              Tel. no. _____

Any other information _____

_____

_____

_____

Note: details of the applicant's/proposed Manager(s)' qualifications/related experience and employment record for the past ten years should be attached to this application on a separate sheet.

Indicate names and relationships of any children/dependent relatives of the applicant(s) of the home who will also be resident on the premises.

Name	Date of Birth	Relationship
Name	Date of Birth	Relationship
Name	Date of Birth	Relationship
Name	Date of Birth	Relationship
Name	Date of Birth	Relationship
Name	Date of Birth	Relationship

Is any person related to the applicant(s) going to be involved in the day-to-day management of the home and in what capacity? Please give details.

Name _____ Relationship _____

Address _____

Capacity _____

If application is for dual registration

1   State Nursing Home Registration Number

2   Name and address of registering Health Authority

Will any other business be transacted on the same premises as the home? If yes give details.

Please give details of any other private or voluntary home in which the applicant has been employed, or has or has had an interest.

Has/ Have the applicant(s) or any other person to be employed in any capacity in the home been convicted of any offence or been subject to any warnings/ de-registration procedures with any other registering authority? If so give details.

References to support this application for registration. Names and addresses of four referees of the applicant(s) (one of whom should be a current or recent employer).

1

2

3

4

5   Name and address of bankers willing to provide financial references.

Note: Where applicants have owned or managed a private or voluntary home in another area a reference should also be obtained from the registering authority.

Names and addresses of four referees for proposed manager (one of whom should be current or recent employer).

1

2

3

4

Section 2   Staffing

Excluding the owners/ manager(s) of the home please give details of proposed staffing:

1	Number of full-time care staff	@	hours per week
2	Number of part-time care staff	@	hours per week
3	Number of domestic staff	@	hours per week
4	Number of cooks	@	hours per week
5	Number of gardeners/ maintenance	@	hours per week
6	Number of resident staff		

Give details of number of qualified staff
Number

Qualifications

Employment Legislation and Health and Safety at Work Act 1974/ 5

Note: Owner and Manager(s) of homes should be able to provide the Registering Authority with samples of job descriptions/ contracts of employment and written statements to staff on Health and Safety at Work.

Section 3   The premises and accommodation to be provided

Description of premises: Please attach site plans of interior design of property giving details of the dimensions of all rooms intended for residents' use, also indicating owners'/ staff private accommodation.

Location of premises (please circle)

City centre	Urban	Within five miles radius of city boundary
Town centre	Within two mile radius of town centre	
Village centre	Within two mile radius of village centre	
Rural isolated	Close to Post Office	shops

Type of property (please circle)

Detached	Semi-detached	Terraced

Approximate date of construction

Roof

Tiles	Slate	Thatch	Flat roof

Facilities

Cavity wall insulation	Double glazing	Main drainage	Septic tank
Gas	Electricity	Bulk Calor gas supply	Solid fuel

Has electrical wiring been checked?   Yes/ No

Details of accommodation for residents' use

No. of	Ground floor	First floor	Second floor
Bathrooms			
Separate WCs			
Showers			
Single bedrooms			
Double bedrooms			

Indicate the number of rooms with en-suite wc/ bathroom facilities

Indicate the number of rooms with space designed to facilitate provision or preparation of drinks/ snack meals and for residents to fully furnish themselves.

Indicate the number of communal rooms

Lounge and sitting	Number	Floor No.
Dining	Number	Floor No.

Indicate the number of rooms with telephone	TV points

Other accommodation (Please circle)

Office/ interview room	Games/ playroom	Sluice room
Rehabilitation flat	Medical treatment room	Guest room for relatives
Workshop	Staff room	or friends
Sick room	Bar	
Reading/ quiet room	Utility room	

Indicate area/ acreage of grounds

Additional out-door facilities (Please circle)

Lawned area for residents' use		Patio area
Playing field	Swimming pool	Tennis court
Bowling green	Greenhouse	Slides/ climbing frame

Opportunities for residents to pursue horticultural/ gardening interests.

Please give information on type/ model of emergency call system.

State if installed in all rooms to be used by residents— including bathrooms/ wcs.   Yes/ No

Indicate provision of any additional adaptations to the premises to assist the physically disabled.

Chair lift	Shaft lift	Hoists
Special bath	Grab rails in bathrooms/ wcs	Adapted telephones
Loop system for the deaf	Ramps for wheelchairs	

Where will drugs/ dangerous drugs cupboard be sited?

Section 4 Health and social care

If home is to accommodate children will educational facilities
be provided on premises?   Yes/ No

What arrangements have been made for health care provision?

1 General practitioner

2 Chiropody

3 Dental care

4 Optician

5 Physiotherapist

6 Occupational therapist

7 Speech therapist

8 Nursing care for minor ailments

9 Psychologist

What arrangements have been made to meet residents' spiritual needs?

What arrangements have been made regarding provision of advice to residents
over financial/ legal matters?

What arrangements have been made regarding residents' personal laundry—
indicating if this is included in weekly accommodation charge?

What are the arrangements for insurance cover of the home? Indicate whether
residents' own furniture/effects are covered by policy:

Name and address of insurance company

Details of other amenities to be provided:

Television	Radio	
Periodicals/ newspapers	Library	Large-print books
Visiting hairdresser	Visits to club/ day centre	Shopping expeditions
Attendance at training centre	Special school	Day school
Participation in adult education	Work centre	Minibus

Provision of meals and special diets:
Attach a proposed two-week menu plan to cover breakfast—lunch—high tea/
dinner.

State the hours between which meals are normally served.

Section 5   Additional registration requirements

Note: the registering authority should have written approval for the following if applicable.

City/ District Council planning approval for a 'Change of Use' to a residential home.

Planning consent no.   Date obtained

City/ District Environmental Health Officer responsible for approving premises under Food Hygiene (General) Regulations 1970 and Health and Safety at Work Act 1974

Name of officer

Address

                                      Tel no.

Name and address of Fire Prevention Officer responsible for approving premises:

Name of officer

Address

                                      Tel no.

If application is for a home which includes children, name and address of GP/ Medical Officer responsible for medical examinations:

Name

Address

                                      Tel no.

Please attach to this application a copy of the home's prospectus/ brochure, the residents' conditions of residence and proposed scale of charges.

Please supply a medical report from the applicant's general practitioner on present state of health.

Any additional information

Certificate of applicant(s)

I/ We certify that the information given in this application for registration is to the best of my/ our knowledge and belief correct and complete and I/ we agree to comply with the registration requirements specified in the Guide to Registration.

Signed

Signed

Date

Annexe 3 Model 2 Homes registration: Formal review/ inspection check list

A suggested model for use by Registration Officers under the Registered Homes Act 1984.

Section 1 | **Residents**

1 Number of residents in residence at time of visit.
2 Total number of deaths in establishment since last review of residents under the age of 65.
3 Number of residents supported by DHSS.
4 Number of residents supported by registering authority.
5 Number of residents supported by other authorities.
6 Amount of grant support per resident.
7 Current weekly inclusive charge of home.
8 Any additional charges.
9 Number of vacancies.
10 For homes accommodating children—how many children are:—
a Subject to care orders.
b Not in care.
11 How often are formal reviews held in the home on each child and resident jointly with a social worker and a parent or relative?
12 Information on frequency of visits by social workers other than at formal reviews.

Section 2 | **Record keeping**

1 Are records kept on each child/resident and were these seen during the inspection?
2 Is a record kept of the name and address of the care/placing authority and is there confirmation that notification of a child's placement was sent to the District Health Authority, the Child Health Service and local Education Authority?
3 Are relevant sections of the Mental Health Act 1983 and social worker recorded?
4 Probation officer responsible in case of probation supervision order?
5 Are current records kept on sanctions applied to control behaviour?
6 Are records kept to provide a receipt for personal allowance allocation—especially for children and mentally handicapped people?

7 Are there current health records on each resident which include details of allocation of medication?

8 Is a record kept of current menu plan/ rota?

9 Are there current records on all staff employed in the home and were staff rotas inspected?

10 Are current records kept on fire alarm tests and fire safety practice? Is there evidence that all staff have received instruction on fire drill and health and safety requirements?

11 Is there a record book kept to record accidents and events of importance?

Section 3   Health and social care

1 Do residents have a choice of doctor?

2 If one practice/ surgery provides medical cover—does the GP call when requested, on routine/liaison visits, weekly fortnightly?

3 Which member of staff has responsibility for the supervision and recording of medication and for the safety, handling and disposal of drugs?

4 Are residents who are capable encouraged to manage their own medication?

5 Number of residents currently in general/ psychiatric hospital?

6 Number of residents incontinent/ doubly incontinent?

7 How many residents were temporarily confined to bed at the time of visit and required constant attention throughout the day and night?

8 Does the community nurse/ psychiatric nurse call?

9 Does the District Health Authority or SSD provide supplies and aids for residents who are incontinent?

10 How are hairdressing services arranged?

11 How are chiropody, dental, ophthalmic, physiotherapy etc services provided? In what form?

12 Is occupational therapy provided and are residents encouraged to pursue individual hobbies/ interests?

13 How many residents have minimal contact with relatives/ friends and are there suitable facilities for these people to be seen in private when they visit the home? Has the SSD been informed about children who have not been visited?

14 How are residents' religious needs being catered for/ which religious denominations arrange regular visits to house bound residents?

15 Are voluntary workers/ visitors encouraged to visit the residents?

16 Do residents receive visits from specialist social workers for the deaf, blind, etc?

Section 4   Community links

1 How many residents regularly receive special services outside the home at:—
  a Adult training centres
  b Special school
  c Day hospital
  d Day centre
  e Sheltered workshops
  f Adult literacy classes
2 How many residents attend activities outside the home?
3 What transport facilities are available for residents?
4 Are communal entertainments/outings organised on a regular basis?

Section 5   Staffing of home

1 How many staff vacancies?
2 Has there been an unusually high turnover of staff since last review?
3 Are staff meetings held on a regular basis?
4 Are there any current staff disputes?
5 How many staff are attending training courses *full* or *part time*?
6 Relevant information on any relatives of proprietor/manager of the home who may be assisting in the care of residents.

Section 6   Catering facilities

1 What are the arrangements for meal times?
2 Do residents have a sufficiently wide choice of menu or of certain foods without extra charge?
3 Are residents requiring special medical diets being catered for?
4 Are residents' religious/cultural food preferences respected?
5 Can residents have their meals in their own rooms?
6 Are there facilities for residents to prepare their own snacks/hot drinks?

Section 7   The premises

1 Decorative order and standard of furnishings.
2 Any repairs/extensions pending.
3 Emergency call system checked.
4 Fire prevention system satisfactory.
5 Central heating system satisfactory.
6 Review of special accommodation facilities, i.e. rehabilitation flat etc.
7 Kitchen and laundry facilities satisfactory.

8 General upkeep of exterior of property and gardens.

9 Comment on general hygiene/ odour control.

Section 8

Management of the home

1 Review of informal visits made throughout the year t registration staff.

2 Review of any complaints about management/ standards home and action taken.

3 If proprietor lives away from the premises does he appointee visit monthly?

4 Are original terms and conditions of registration still beir complied with?

5 Are there likely to be any changes in the managemer structure of the home during the next twelve months. e. change of ownership?

Note

Following each formal review a report/ letter must be ser to the Proprietor and Manager highlighting any major poin discussed during the registration officer's visit and notin any changes in the conditions of registration, requests for action.

Annexe 4 Behaviour modification

Residents' behaviour will be influenced or 'modified' by many factors, some of which may be introduced deliberately, others of which will coincidentally bring about change. Staff should treat residents with the utmost regard for dignity, privacy and individuality. A care programme designed with these points in mind rarely causes problems in a moral or ethical sense, although in broad terms this may be called behaviour modification.

Difficulty or anxiety arises when a specific piece of bad or socially unacceptable behaviour requires a special programme with some kind of sanction or penalty applied if the client does not respond. There is often misunderstanding about the word 'sanction' when used in connection with behaviour modification. Sanctions may be 'positive', i.e. something which the client will like or enjoy, or 'negative', i.e. something the client dislikes or finds unpleasant. In order to avoid misunderstanding the 'negative sanction' is described throughout the rest of this section as a 'penalty'. The following guidance is intended to clarify this matter and relates to this second definition only, i.e. the kind of special programme which may be appropriate for an individual resident and which entails the use of penalties. Where the programme depends on positive responses such as encouragement, praise, reassurance, additional attention, etc. from staff, no difficulty would be anticipated.

a   Specific behaviour modification programmes must always be drawn up by somebody with the appropriate professional skills and experience. This will usually be a clinical or educational psychologist or a consultant psychiatrist.

b   Any such specific programme should be written down in detail by the person compiling it and used only for the resident for whom it is designed, and never transferred to another resident however similar his behaviour pattern might seem. The purpose of any programme should be explained to the resident and his consent to participation in it obtained.

c   Certain penalties are excluded as being contrary to law. These include physical chastisement of adults, locking residents in isolation, depriving them of food or sleep as a punishment. Any action which would be illegal when applied to a non-resident is also forbidden. An example of this would be the bodily searching of an adult without his permission.

d   Other penalties may be permissible in the context of a specifically designed programme. Examples could be removing the resident from a group, not permitting him to join in a certain activity, not replacing food which the resident has thrown away. This is not the same as depriving the resident of a meal as a punishment for some unconnected piece of behaviour; it is an illustration of a client depriving himself of food within a pattern of behaviour which a special programme is designed to change.

e   Where the resident is fully competent intellectually to understand the implications of a penalty and to give informed consent to the application, there should be no difficulty in implementing that particular programme. However when a resident is not competent to so agree, considerable caution would need to be exercised. In law, unless the resident is under control via certain sections of the Mental Health Act 1983, nobody has the requisite authority to impose treatment of this nature against the resident's will.

Annexe 5 Calculation of staff ratios and hours

One possible method for calculating staffing, given in brief below, is described more fully in *Staffing ratios in residential establishments,* published by the Residential Care Association (now known as the Social Care Association).

The following hours per resident per annum are required:

Mentally ill	416
Low dependency mentally handicapped adults	312
High dependency mentally handicapped adults	676
Physically handicapped adults	780
Elderly physically dependent	572
Elderly mentally infirm	676

On this basis a home for 30 elderly mentally infirm residents would require $30 \times 676 = 20{,}280$ hours of care and managerial time per annum. A hostel for 10 physically handicapped adults would need $10 \times 780 = 7{,}800$ hours. These figures would apply unless minimum cover exceeded the calculated total.

No research-based figures are currently available for other groups such as the less dependent elderly, who constitute a large proportion of the residents in voluntary and private homes, and estimates will have to be made in calculating requirements.

In the two examples above, the staffing would be calculated by dividing the client care hours required by the hours staff can provide (generally, 1,500 hours per person per year). The thirty-place home for the elderly mentally infirm would require $20{,}280 \div 1{,}500 = 13.5$ full-time equivalent staff. The hostel for physically handicapped adults would need $7{,}800 \div 1{,}500 = 5.2$ full-time equivalent staff; since this is below the minimum cover requirement for two staff on duty, amounting to a need for 7.0 staff, the minimum would be applied.

Annexe 6 Sources of evidence, information and advice

The following organisations and individuals gave evidence and we acknowledge their help with appreciation.

Organisations that provided additional comments, oral evidence or took part in discussions are denoted in bold italic type.

We also wish to thank many other people, whose names do not appear below, who answered our questions or contributed informally at various stages in the preparation of this document.

Local Authorities' Social Services Departments:

Metropolitan and London boroughs
Barnet, Bexley, Bradford, Bromley, Bury, Lambeth, Newham, Rotherham, Sefton, Wandsworth.

County councils
Avon, Bedfordshire, Cambridgeshire, Cheshire, Clwyd, Devon, Dorset, Durham, Eastern Health and Social Services Board — Belfast, *East Sussex*, Essex, Gloucestershire, Hampshire, Isle of Wight, Lancashire, Lincolnshire, Lothian, Norfolk, North Yorkshire, Nottinghamshire, South Glamorgan, Warwickshire, West Sussex, Wiltshire.

National Government Departments:

Department of Health and Social Security
Department of Health and Social Services, N. Ireland
Department of the Environment
Department of Education and Science
The Housing Corporation

Community Health Councils:
Aberconwy, Bath, Bexley, Brighton, Cambridge, Central Manchester, Clwyd South, Coventry, East Cumbria, East Hertfordshire, Frenchay, Hampstead, Harrow, Hull, Lancaster, Lincolnshire North, Manchester North, Merton and Sutton, Newham, North Bedfordshire, North East Essex, North East Yorkshire, North Gwent, Peterborough, Plymouth, Somerset, South Cumbria, South East Kent, South Tyneside, South Warwickshire, Southend, Wakefield (Western), West Birmingham, West Essex, West Lancashire, Winchester and Central Hampshire, Worcester, York.

Health authorities:
National Association of Health Authorities — Working Party on Private Nursing Homes, Oxfordshire Health Authority

Registered Rest Homes Associations:
National Confederation of Registered Rest Homes Associations, Hampshire, Kent, Lincolnshire and South Humberside, Southport, Suffolk, West Sussex.

Private and voluntary residential care homes:	Ashleigh Rest Home, Tunbridge Wells; Bradfield Place, Nr. Manningtree; Bryony Home, Birmingham; Cecil Houses, Kew; Convent of the Holy Family, Bromley; Dr. French Memorial Home, London N12; The Elms, Llandudno; Fern Hill, Burnley; Fairfield, Oxford; Foundation of Edward Storey, Cambridge; Franjos, Dymchurch; Greylands, Morecambe; Halsey House, London WC1; The Haven Rest Home, Bournemouth; Heatherlea House, Woodhall Spa; Hollybank, Kenley; The Mayflowers, Colwyn Bay; National Westminster Staff Foundation — Oldroyd House, Canterbury; Olton Grange, Solihull; Parkview, London SE19; Red House, Milton Keynes; Rest Home for the Elderly, Leigh-on-Sea; Rochester House, Ross-on-Wye; Royal Star and Garter Home for Disabled Sailors, Soldiers and Airmen, Richmond, Surrey; St. Joseph's Home, Warrenpoint; St. Margaret's Private Nursing Home, Hythe; St. Mary's House, Bungay; Sceats Memorial Eventide Home, Gloucester; Senior Citizens Housing Society Ltd. — Eastwood, London N3; The Squirrels, Poole; Templeton, London SW16; Zetland Court, Bournemouth.
Professional bodies and voluntary organisations:	Abbeyfield Morecambe and Heysham Society; Abbeyfield Society; Age Concern, Bromley; *Age Concern, England; Association of Charity Officers; Association of County Councils; Association of Directors of Social Services;* Association of Directors of Social Work; *Association of Metropolitan Authorities;* Association of Residential Communities for the Retarded; Association for Residential Mental Care; Bristol Old People's Welfare Inc.; *British Association of Social Workers;* British Geriatrics Society; The Campaign for Mentally Handicapped People; *Centre for Policy on Ageing;* Centre on Environment for the Handicapped; *Children's Legal Centre;* Church of England Pensions Board; Council for the Education and Training of Health Visitors; Counsel and Care for the Elderly; Deal Old People's Housing Society Ltd.; Royal College of Physicians, Faculty of Community Medicine; *Federation of Alcoholic Rehabilitation Establishments;* Gold Hill Housing Association; Gospel Standard Bethesda Fund; Health Visitors Association; Help the Aged Housing Appeal; Jewish Welfare Board; *King's Fund Centre;* Leonard Cheshire Foundation; London Boroughs Children's Regional Planning Committee; MENCAP (National Society for Mentally Handicapped Children and Adults); Methodist Homes for the Aged; *MIND (National Association for Mental Health);* Mutual Aid Homes; Pharmaceutical Society of Great Britain; *Registered Nursing Homes Association; Residential Care Association (renamed Social Care Association);* Richmond upon Thames Churches Housing Trust Ltd.; Royal College of General Practitioners; Royal College of Nursing; Royal College of Psychiatrists; *Royal National Institute for the Blind; Royal National Institute for the Deaf;* Royal United Kingdom

Beneficent Association; Scottish Health Education Group; *Standing Conference on Drug Abuse;* Sue Ryder Foundation, *West of England Friends Housing Society Ltd.;* Worthing Are. Guild for Voluntary Service.

Members of professions, universities and colleges:	Mrs. E. M. Crawford (Nursing Officer), Mrs. F. A. Hanes (District Dietitian), Miss M. Marshall (Lecturer in Social Sciences), Mrs. E. Palmer (Nursing Officer), Dr. R. M. Philpott (Consultant Psychogeriatrician), Dr. S. Peace (Research Fellow), Dr. G. Roberts (Senior Lecturer in Social Policy), Miss M. Soufflet (Chiropodist).
Members of the public:	Dr. M. S. Chesters, Mrs. M. Diggle, Miss M. Henner, Mr. D. Jarvis, Mrs. F. Molyneux, Ms. G. V. Pratt, Miss E. F. Whitney.
Establishments visited:	Cheshire Home, Cardiff; Hales House, Norfolk; Hill Homes, London; Phoenix House, London; Richmond Fellowship, London and Surrey.